Katterfelto
prince of puff

To Norman & Vera
with love
David

David Paton-Williams

Katterfelto
prince of puff

Matador
9 De Montfort Mews
Leicester LE1 7FW, UK
Tel: (+44) 116 255 9311 / 9312
Email: books@troubador.co.uk
Web: www.troubador.co.uk/matador

ISBN 978-1906510-916

A Cataloguing-in-Publication (CIP) catalogue record for this book
is available from the British Library.

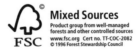

Mixed Sources
Product group from well-managed
forests and other controlled sources
www.fsc.org Cert no. TT-COC-2082
© 1996 Forest Stewardship Council

Typeset in 11pt Stempel Garamond by Troubador Publishing Ltd, Leicester, UK
Printed in the UK by The Cromwell Press Ltd, Trowbridge, Wilts, UK

Matador is an imprint of Troubador Publishing Ltd

To Jenny, Edward and George
For sharing the journey

CONTENTS

LIST OF ILLUSTRATIONS

PREFACE

Walk into any ancient church and you are surrounded by stories. The memorials, the effigies and the architecture itself, all tell the history of a community. They provide a glimpse of the people and values that have shaped it. The church of St Gregory in Bedale is no exception. This ancient North Yorkshire building tells tales of Viking Christians and raiding Scots, as well as of the quiet, domesticated lives of gentry and commoner. However, one of its greatest tales is not told by the church itself. For under the floor, hidden from view near the communion rail, lies something of a mystery.

Buried there are the bones of a man. He was not a resident of the town, nor even a native of these shores and yet his remains lie in a place of privilege granted only to the few. Who was he? How did he come to lie here and why was he granted such an honour?

If you had stood at his grave two hundred years ago you would have read the following epitaph: "Christian William Anthony Katterfelto, Doctor in Philosophy, died November 15th 1799, aged 56 years".[1] Beyond the parish boundaries the general public may well have felt some surprise, even shock, had it been known where he was buried. To many he was worthy of no such honour, having, they thought, defrauded much of the nation. Some may even have believed that he had supped with the devil. To himself, Katterfelto was a brilliant natural philosopher, an ingenious inventor, a skilful magician, a philanthropic purveyor of medicines, a fearless explorer and much else besides. To his detractors (and he accumulated many) he was a pompous buffoon and a money-grabbing one at that. From our own vantage point, the least we can say is that he was a showman, perhaps one of the greatest entertainers of the eighteenth century.

Like his grave, much of the truth about who Katterfelto really was is also hidden. It lies behind a flamboyant self-image that he projected in his publicity and his performances. For he has rarely been surpassed in the art of self-promotion. He was the eighteenth century king of spin, or, in the language of the day, the "prince of puff". Two decades of extravagant, even outrageous, advertisements made him a household name throughout the land. Fortunately, this need for publicity - a need that was driven as much by his own personality as by the requirements of his profession - has left behind a trail. It can be followed through the pages of the ever-growing number of newspapers that were springing up around Britain. These papers not only help to tell Katterfelto's story but also the story of life in Britain during the last quarter of the eighteenth century.

Over a hundred years before, Dryden had written of a "year of wonders". Following in the footsteps of Katterfelto leads us back into an age of wonders: wonders of science, medicine, exploration and sheer entertainment. Katterfelto did his best to capitalise on these and to place himself at the centre of many of them. He was determined to become the greatest wonder of them all: "that wonderful wonder, the great Katterfelto".[2]

----

[1] Hird's Annals of Bedale, ed. Lesley Lewis, North Yorkshire County Council, 1975, page 223

[2] The Grand Consultation, George Canning

CHAPTER 1

A WANDERING STAR

"And Katterfelto with his hair on end
At his own wonders, wondering for his bread!"
William Cowper, "The Task", book 4, 1785

The quayside at Hull was buzzing as usual. It was Thursday 26ᵗʰ September 1776 and a fleet of barges had made its way down a growing network of navigable rivers and canals to one of England's four largest ports. They had brought Cheshire cheeses, Staffordshire earthenware, Derbyshire lead, cloth from Lancashire and wool from Yorkshire. Now the exports of northern England were being stowed into the holds of ships that would soon set sail for the continent. Meanwhile, vessels from Petersburg, Danzig and the other Baltic ports, as well as two newly arrived from Amsterdam, were being unloaded by the stevedores. Most of their cargo was heading for Britain's dockyards to help build its merchant and military fleets: timber from Russian firs, pitch and tar, bundles of flax for sails, hemp, iron, linseed, and even brush-bristles were all making their way down onto the quayside.[1] Nearby on the docks stood a few passengers who had made the journey across the North Sea. They carried no passports and no immigration officials were there to meet them; not until 1793, with a rising tide of refugees fleeing revolutionary France, would Britain begin keeping records of those entering the country.

Among the human cargo stepping onto British soil that day was a young German family. A thin man, about 5'10" tall and in his early thirties, was standing beside his wife who was clearly in the last stages of pregnancy. Next to them their six-year old daughter sat playing with a black kitten. The attention of the parents was focussed on the men who were unloading a set of well-made boxes of all shapes and sizes from one of the ships. Not before all these containers had been

1

carefully reloaded onto a large horse-drawn wagon would the three of them leave the docks. The Katterfelto family - William, Martha and Mary - had arrived.

Some ten days later Mr. Katterfelto walked into the office of the York Courant and, in a thick German accent, dictated an advertisement for the paper's next edition. It duly appeared on Tuesday 8th October and is the earliest surviving example of several hundreds which were published by him in Britain over the next twenty-three years:

> On the 26th of September – arrived at Hull where he has ever since performed in the Concert-Room with universal Applause, a Son of Col. KATTERFELTO of the famous Prussian Regiment of Death-Head Hussars, Professor of Natural Philosophy, Mathematics, Astronomy, Geography, Fortification, Navigation etc. For 15 years past he has travelled thro' most Parts of Europe, and spent a considerable Fortune, purposely to improve himself in Philosophy and Mathematics, and has finished a curious Apparatus for his own Amusement, and for the Instruction of the Public. – He will exhibit in Nicholson's Great Room, Coney-Street York, To-morrow Evening (Oct.9) and every Evening this Week. The Doors will be opened at Six, and the Performance to begin at Seven. Admittance to the three front Seats 2s each, back Seats 1s only. – His various astonishing Performances are fully expressed in Hand-Bills which will be delivered this Day. – He goes from this City to Leeds, Wakefield, Halifax etc.[2]

By the standards of most of Katterfelto's later publicity material this advert is fairly low-key, even modest. However, it offers us a tantalising hint of his life-story so far. Putting it together with other remarks that he makes about himself over the next few years we get the following, pretty impressive, curriculum vitae prior to his arrival in Britain. He was a Prussian, from Berlin,[3] who had been born into a highly successful military family. His father had been the Colonel of the elite and exotically named Death's Head Hussars and his uncle had held an even more exalted rank:

> The late General Katterfelto, his uncle, and the late Colonel Katterfelto, his father, were two favourites last war of the King of Prussia, as they took many thousand prisoners.[4]

The war in question was the Seven Years War (1756-1763). The young Katterfelto had also fought in it, rising like his father to the rank of Colonel, while his brother served as a Captain in the same regiment of hussars as his father.[5] Even so, the war had not been an unmitigated success for the Katterfeltos. This became clear when a certain French nobleman was visiting London in 1782:

> *The reason of Comte De Grasse taking such great notice of Mr KATTERFELTO is because Comte De Grasse took his father and him prisoner when the former was Colonel of the Death's Head Hussars, belonging to the King of Prussia, at the battle of Schwerein, in the year 1759.*[6]

After the war Katterfelto left the army and began his journeys around Europe. He travelled in order to learn and to teach, sharing with his audiences the wonders of the physical universe, as well as giving them guidance on the moral and spiritual path of life. Over the next fifteen years he acquired the title of Professor in a variety of subjects and exhibited at most of Europe's Universities[7] and Courts. His audiences included the "Empress of Russia, the Queen of Hungary, the Kings of Prussia, Sweden, Denmark and Poland".[8] To have exhibited in Petersburg (where he performed for Catherine the Great on the occasion of her birthday in 1768),[9] Vienna, Berlin, Stockholm, Copenhagen and Warsaw meant that Katterfelto had performed in the imperial and royal capitals of the whole of central, northern and eastern Europe, with the exception of the Ottoman Empire. (He had even found time to perform in Paris and Dresden.)[10]

Such then was the pedigree of the man. Or rather, such was the image he wanted to present of himself. Doubts are raised at just about every point of the story. Take his military record. To begin with, his capture at the Battle of Schwerein could not have happened for one very simple reason: there was no such battle. In fact, the Seven Years War didn't even come close to this area of northern Germany. Nor could the Comte de Grasse possibly have taken Katterfelto and his father prisoner in a land battle, because the Count was actually in the navy. As for Katterfelto's rank of Colonel: at the end of the war he was no more than about twenty years old. He must have been a soldier of truly exceptional ability to have risen to such an exalted rank at so tender an age.

Then there are the Death's Head Hussars, so named after the skull that decorated their headgear. These were the most dashing of all the Prussian cavalry regiments and their officers were invariably drawn from the upper echelons of the nobility. For his father to have been their commanding officer would have been an honour indeed. So then, not quite the social background that we might expect of a travelling entertainer-cum-lecturer. Katterfelto certainly became famous for the Death's Head Hussar officer's hat and the immense (and rusty) sword that he sported on stage. These, he claimed, had been worn by his grandfather the General, "when he took 30,000 prisoners."[11] However, Hussars were light cavalry whose swords were only arm-length sabres. So were the cap and sword genuine family memorabilia? Or had he simply picked them up on his travels in post-war Germany as handy props for the creation of a stage persona? No doubt the aura surrounding the recently successful Prussian army served him well as he tried to establish his reputation among the ladies and gentlemen of English society. However, once he had made a name for himself in London during the early 1780s, he was happy to let his family origins drop out of his publicity almost completely. From then on it seems that he no longer needed to trade on a dubious military background.

To his stage persona we can even add his name, because one thing is for sure: "Katterfelto" isn't a German name. On the other hand "Katterfelt" is. Its roots (in a variety of spellings)[12] lie around the small village of Catterfeld in central Germany. This area didn't become part of Prussia until the nineteenth century but by the mid-seventeen hundreds the family name had already spread to other German states. So our hero may well have been a Prussian. However, wherever he had come from, given that Prussia was one of the rising stars among the European nations at the time, it would certainly have suited him to bask in some of its reflected glory. As we shall see, Katterfelto was never a man to let the facts get in the way of a good story.

It seems then, that following in the footsteps of many a travelling quack and conjuror, Katterfelto's autobiography was largely a fiction. What we are able to say is that he was undoubtedly of German origin; that (based on his gravestone) he was born in about 1743; and that in his late teens or early twenties he had begun travelling around Europe. He usually dates the start of these journeys to the period of 1763-5, (although occasional references put it as early as 1760).[13] This more or less coincides with the end of the Seven Years War. Peace on the Continent meant that large numbers of men now had to find new employment but there was also a far greater freedom of movement right across Europe. Along with many other entertainers, Katterfelto took full advantage of it.

Wherever his journeys may have taken him, over the years he certainly gained a reasonable amount of scientific understanding, developed considerable skills as a conjuror and acquired a competency in English that, for all the jingoistic mockery of it, was sufficient for him to perform in a foreign land for many years. Add to this an honorary "professorship" and a single vowel to the end of his name and, hey presto: the great Katterfelto was born. Katterfelto - now there was a name to conjure with!

The end of the war also meant that Britain was open to Continental performers, who grasped the opportunity with both hands. When Katterfelto brought his family across the North Sea in September 1776 he was joining in this peace dividend for entertainers. Armed with his stage name and persona, Katterfelto and family sailed for Hull (the main point of arrival for ships from north east Europe) and set out to captivate the great British public.

From the first advertisement in York we can see something of his strategy. He would set himself up in a well-to-do part of town (provided that the funds were available and that the town was in fact well-to-do.) He would then invest two or three shillings a time in the local paper, announcing that here was a man of great learning and invention: an educator and entertainer, whose exhibitions and performances had created widespread astonishment and acclaim wherever he had been. Provincial newspapers were on the increase and would serve Katterfelto well in large towns and cities. Almost every county had its own paper and the few exceptions were covered by papers from neighbouring shires. However, despite their widening circulation, he needed other ways to publicise himself. So he backed up the adverts with handbills available at his venues, distributed in the streets or posted on walls. He also made use of the tried and tested method of supposedly unsolicited tributes.

These began to appear a week after he had announced his arrival in York. The next edition of the Courant carried a poem headed "Hull, September 30th", purporting to have been "Wrote extempore on seeing Mr KATTERFELTO's Great Exhibition":

His Ship beyond Description lies,
When well observ'd by curious Eyes;
The Guns, no thicker than a Straw,
Go off by philosophic Law.

5

Without the Help of Match or Fire,
Which all applaud, and some admire.
His Fountain plays both Fire and Water,
Which entertains, and causes Laughter.
By virtue of his Magic Skill
He makes an Hour-Glass stand still,
And run again in half a Minute,
As fast as if the Devil was in it.
By tricks with Figures and with Letters,
He amuses and instructs his Betters.
By his great Art you're next a Trial,
When he shews his amazing Dial,
And by th' Electrical Machine
He shews what ne'er before was seen,
And by the Difference of eyes
He pleases them with great Surprize,
And in the Art of Gunnery
Surprises them uncommonly,
And in the Plaincessit Art
He shews each Lady her Sweetheart,
And by the Caprimandick Noughts
Discovers every Persons Thoughts.
His little Dutchman, I protest,
Surpris'd me more than all the rest.
And in Dexterity of Hand,
He makes a most delightful End.

Over the years Katterfelto published many such tributes, supposedly written by various "members of the audience". Often the poems were reprinted in different papers, each time presented as being hot off the press. Occasionally they were even honoured with a place in "Poet's Corner", which was a regular feature on the back page of many papers. Sadly, the offerings were usually little better than this one, and sometimes worse. However, the poems do help to piece together details of his performances.

Here, in this first offering, we glimpse the way that Katterfelto would continually bring together conjuring and science to both amuse and instruct his audience, presenting himself not merely as an entertainer but also as a philosopher. In eighteenth century Britain there was a great hunger for learning about the discoveries of "natural philosophy", as the science of the day was usually called.

Many of these new insights lent themselves to being illustrated by some spectacular demonstrations, making it an age when adult education and entertainment went hand in hand. As a result it was a time well-suited to the likes of Katterfelto. On this particular evening in York, he had included an "Electrical Machine" and an "amazing Dial" to illustrate his scientific points; had lectured on optics ("the Difference of eyes"); and had used small pieces of phosphorus to ignite the cannons on his model ship. He had then rounded off the evening with such magical deceptions as stopping and starting an hourglass, a dramatic gun trick and a mind-reading act.

At the end of the York poem Katterfelto announced that his "curious Performances" would be exhibited for another week before he moved on to pastures new. However, his departure was slightly delayed: the reason being that the following day his wife gave birth to a baby boy. Frederick William Katterfelto was christened on Sunday 27th October 1776 at St Michael-le-Belfry Church, in the same font as one Guido Fawkes two centuries before. The parish registers give the names of the boy's parents as William and "Mathai" (a form of Martha) with the father having no profession other than being "a Prussian".

The pause for the birth and baptism of his son seems to have been no longer than it needed to be. There was no paternity leave for travelling entertainers in the eighteenth century; nor was there much time for their wives to recover. Two days after the service, and less than a fortnight after the birth, a third and final advert appeared in the Courant. It announced that the Colonel's son had "Yesterday arrived at Leeds from York" (though no advert appears in the Leeds papers at the time) and made it clear to the readers that he was on a mission to educate the inhabitants of this fast expanding industrial town:

His Lectures and surprising Experiments are Philosophical, Mathematical, Optical, Magnetical, Electrical, Physical, Chemical, Pneumatic, Hydraulic, Perotic, Hydrostatic, Stenographic, Pollengestic, and Caprimandic Arts.[14]

What a list! Some words defy definition, and his thick accent often made it even harder for newspaper clerks to know how to spell some of them. Take the word "Pollengistic". This may be a version of "Palingenesy", which a book of magic tricks at the time described as making images appear in a glass jar, such as an artificial rose or "the image of a deceased Person".[15] (The "Plaincessit Art" of his earlier poem, which showed ladies their sweethearts, was possibly yet another spelling of a similar illusion.)

Then there is "Caprimandic". Ten years earlier a French conjuror called Comus had advertised "an operation of caperomancy" and Katterfelto was following suit.[16] Although the spelling varied over the years, the word seems to hint mischievously at the black arts. It suggests divination ("-mancy") by means of the goat (as in Capri-corn). And who was often pictured in goat-like form but Old Nick himself? Did Katterfelto stand inside a magic circle - the "Caprimandick Nought" of his poem - to "discover every person's thoughts"? Was he suggesting that his mind-reading powers came from a more sinister source than mere conjuring? He certainly played on this idea in years to come.

Katterfelto's affection for grand words was something he was to become both famous and ridiculed for. For example, in 1784, theatregoers at Whitby were treated to a farce that included "The fatal Overthrow of Abobecocracoponocopifficacokatterfelto, King of the Antipodeans."[17] However, this sort of elaborate and pompous phraseology was common among his peers in the world of conjuring, many of whom had already been mocked by John "Orator" Henley. Henley was a non-conformist minister who, from the 1720's to 1740's, became the first person in England to make widespread use of the medium of newspaper advertisements. Drawing on the verbal techniques of conjurors and fortune-tellers, he produced hundreds of nonsensical adverts offering instruction in, for example, the "Mettallurgic, Typographic, Gnomonic, Scenographic, Isotropic, Biantic, Theeutic, Ixeutic, Halieutic, Cynegetic arts of the Ancients and Moderns".[18]

Katterfelto could not have known Henley, who had died twenty years before the German arrived in Britain. However, the similarity between their styles may suggest that Katterfelto used an English copywriter to help compose some of his advertisements. This was certainly the conclusion drawn by at least one eyewitness who believed that the mixture of German and English in Katterfelto's shows made them "incoherent exhibitions" and revealed his dependency on a "literary journeyman".[19] Whatever the precise authorship of some of his adverts, over the years to come they were going to make him famous throughout the land.

Following his time in York and Leeds, Katterfelto may have moved on to Wakefield and Halifax as he had planned but his travels in Yorkshire in the late 1770s certainly included a first visit to Bedale. His arrival there was witnessed and remembered by a young boy by the name of Robert Hird. In later life Hird was to become the local shoemaker and he went on to record his childhood memories in a large volume of naïve verse known as the "Annals of Bedale". In these he recounts the day when a stranger arrived in the small market town, with a retinue that now included a young black servant. Together they caused no small stir:

> One day, when playing in the street,
> A waggon we did see,
> And presently we did it meet,
> It quite delighted me.
> The waggon, it was very long,
> And it was cover'd in,
> Beside the horses they were strong,
> We such had seldom seen.
> And more than this I can tell you,
> To us it was delight!
> A fine young Blackamoor to view!
> Most curious was the sight!

The visitors then took up residence in one of the local hostelries, the Black Swan Inn in the main street.

> Next day the black went round the town,
> And often made a stand!
> His trumpet he did blow anon!
> His voice had great command!
> All silence and attention paid,
> To hear him tell his tale,
> And when they'd heard what he had said,
> The boys again did sail!
> What he did say was news all round,
> The gents they must all go!
> Phylosopher, did all astound!
> Doctor Katterfelto!!!
> The great man here was well receiv'd,
> And he did make long stay!
> His art and knowledge they believ'd,
> And when he went away

He was talk'd of for many years,
With greatest memory,
Of him they talk'd, like ancient seers,
But lost all hope to see
That he or waggon again should come
With bird cages hung round!
Phylosophers, no other one,
The road to Bedale found.[20]

(Hird says that this first visit occurred some twenty years before Katterfelto's death in 1799. Katterfelto also visited Yorkshire in 1786-7, but by then he had two servants and his horses were in a sorry state, as we shall see. So we can confidently date his first visit to Bedale sometime between the end of 1776 and 1780.)

If blowing a trumpet was not sufficient to attract people's attention then seemingly the appearance of a young black boy in rural eighteenth century North Yorkshire definitely was. This lad was part of a black population in Britain that has been estimated at between ten to fifteen thousand people.[21] They were spread through many towns and cities although the majority were living in London. Some were freemen and women, working as sailors, in business or as musicians. Among those who were servants, some were paid and could leave their master's employ, although others were still very definitely slaves and treated as property. Wherever Katterfelto had taken on, or bought, his servant, and however he was treated, the boy not only indicated that Katterfelto was a gentleman but also added an exotic fascination to his show, at least in the less cosmopolitan parts of the country, such as Bedale.

We can also see that the folk of this little town had taken Katterfelto to their hearts, believing that a great philosopher had indeed visited them. But then again, according to Hird, they had had little to compare him to. What other roads this particular philosopher found over the next four years is not clear. Towards the end of 1777 he certainly exhibited for a week in Gloucester.[22] However, it is not until 1780 that Katterfelto's trail reappears but then it has a scent strong enough to be followed for the best part of two decades. On the 9th December 1780 the Katterfelto Show arrived in London's West End.[23] It was to have a run of some three and a half years before it toured the provinces again (though he did leave London for six months in the second half of 1781). Over those years the star of the show made his name and, so he said, his fortune.

London, the largest city in the world, was in the throes of urban regeneration, Georgian style. Actually, it was a tale of two cities. Most of the capital's population of close on a million people were crammed into the East End with its poor housing and narrow, dark and badly paved streets. On the other hand, the rich were increasingly escaping from this overcrowding, with its attendant squalor, and moving into the fashionable, open squares and elegant, straight streets that were being built in London's West End. It was a time of opulence in architecture and of sophistication and practicality in urban planning. London's Georgian makeover would eventually include ornate gardens, street lighting and even house numbering.

Expensive shops enabled the fortunate few to equip and decorate their new homes in great style with silks, silver, glass and Wedgwood china, or other fashionable neoclassical ornaments. There were watchmakers, fan stores, confectioners and fruiterers, all helping to make the West End a shopper's paradise. The affluence of this fast emerging consumer society also affected the social life of the city. This began early and finished late. It was vibrant and diverse and was a honey pot that attracted a wide range of entertainers from all over Europe.

It was here in the exciting and rapidly changing West End that Katterfelto set out to establish himself with a sales pitch that was aimed as high as it could go: at "the ladies and gentlemen of Distinction". Looking for a venue, he pulled out all the stops and settled upon the Great Rooms at Spring Gardens. This was one of the best-known and most prestigious locations in London. Formerly a Huguenot Chapel, it included the concert hall that had witnessed Mozart's London debut. Also, until a few years before, it had housed the famous Cox's Museum. James Cox was a celebrated jeweller and metalworker who had designed and made intricate and lavish ornaments, including many automata. The most famous of these was a life-sized silver swan, which preened itself and dipped its beak into the "water" to catch a fish. (It now takes pride of place in the Bowes Museum at Barnard Castle in County Durham.) Cox had exhibited the swan in 1772 and it soon became one of the great attractions of London. However, Cox's financial troubles meant that within a few years he was forced to dispose of his exhibition by lottery.[24] Despite this demise, Spring Gardens remained the place to be seen. So, if it was good enough for Mozart and Cox, then nothing less would do for a philosopher who had enlightened the royalty of Europe (even if later he would move to other London venues.)

Here in the West End the world would learn of Katterfelto's

many "wonders": of illness banished; of magical illusions transcending this-worldly explanations; of his accomplice, the "famous Morocco Black Cat"; of scientific discoveries to rival Isaac Newton; and of pioneering feats of aerial exploration. Here, also, he was ridiculed as an "insolent puffer" whose advertisements would "gibbet him up to posterity as one of the most enterprising imposters that ever made an attack on the pockets of the credulous and unthinking people of this country."[25] Here though, by his relentless publicity campaign, he forced his name into the consciousness of royalty, prime ministers, archbishops and the whole British nation. Eventually he even forced his name into the English language itself.

In London he prospered. He boasted of having been able to purchase a fine new coach and of having earned over £3000, no small fortune in those days. Whatever the true figure may have been, it was certainly more than enough to justify taking into his entourage another servant, or "apprentice" as Katterfelto called him. A fairly detailed, if heavily glossed, account of this new relationship was published in Lincolnshire, during the winter of 1786, when the young man had apparently run away from his master:

On Sunday morning last, between the hours of six and seven o'clock, one of Dr Katterfelto's black boys absconded from him at Grantham, and as he is an apprentice, he therefore gives this notice, that if any person harbours or employs him they will be prosecuted according to law, but if the boy returns, or any person will bring him back, the crime will be forgiven him for this time. He had on when he went away, a great brown coat with white plain buttons, and a little round hat, a black waistcoat and jacket, with little white plain buttons, three rows of buttons on the waistcoat and tassels and shoulder knots on the jacket, a pair of nankeen breeches and boots on. He is about 17 or 18 years of age, middle size, and has a scar on his forehead about half an inch long, is slender made, and has four years to serve to Dr Katterfelto. The boy's name is Thomas Montague, but is liable to change his name; he was christened in St Martin's church, London, before he was bound apprentice to Dr Katterfelto. Any poor person who may have seen the above black boy since last Sunday, and will bring or send word to Dr Katterfelto, now in Newark, so that he may have the said apprentice again, shall be well rewarded for their trouble and all reasonable expenses paid.[26]

A similar notice had appeared some two years earlier while he was still in London. "A little black boy," had run away and could readily be recognised on account of "a little white Spot on his Forehead". He had apparently come from Jamaica, and said of himself that he had been "stolen away from his Father and Mother by a Gunner of a Ship."[27]

These sorts of advertisements, offering rewards for runaway apprentices or slaves, were common in the eighteenth century press. Perhaps Thomas was not a very successful escapee, or perhaps this was all mere puffery, with Katterfelto casting himself in a prosperous yet injured light. Apprentices were indentured at a premium to masters who worked in traditional trades, skilled crafts or professions. So, by calling his servant an apprentice Katterfelto was also laying claim to be viewed as someone of a respectable economic standing.

London certainly served Katterfelto well during his long stay but by the summer of 1784 he had decided that it was time to move on. He gave up on London; or rather London gave up on him. To surrender the settled and relatively comfortable life of the capital for the uncertainties and hardships of the open road suggests that his star was very much on the wane. After years of his "wonders" the London public had finally tired of him once and for all. By now, other entertainments were capturing the imagination of the chattering classes and other new wonders were drawing rich and poor alike to stare in amazement.

So in the middle of July he exhibited for one last time and prepared to leave. Once again the boxes of scientific and magical equipment were stored carefully onto the wagon, along with the rest of the family's possessions. The wagon was hitched up to the horses. The family climbed aboard, together with the servants and what was now a veritable clutter of cats, and off they set. Katterfelto had trailed this move quite heavily, letting it be known that he would "on the 13th July, next, positively set off for St Petersburgh"[28] to perform before "Her Imperial Majesty".[29] In fact, he headed not to the dockyards but east into Essex along the road to Colchester. The road was a long one and it never found its way back to London again.

It took him up through East Anglia, Cambridgeshire, Lincolnshire and back to Yorkshire. It continued on through Durham and Northumberland and up the east coast of Scotland, via Edinburgh at least as far north as Inverness. His path then brought him back down through the Highlands, via Glasgow, to the south west of Scotland. A six-month tour of the Lake District led on through Lancashire and Cheshire to the West Midlands, where he spent over a year in Birmingham. The road then carried him along the Welsh borders from Oswestry to Monmouth and over the River Severn to Gloucester. He wound his way back up through Warwickshire, Derbyshire and Nottinghamshire and as far north as Tyneside, before heading south for a fourth and final visit to the county of Yorkshire where it had all begun. (For a detailed itinerary see the appendix.)

The journey lasted a full fifteen years. It took the Katterfelto family through Britain's fast-developing industrial towns and cities, as well as its countless market towns and rural villages. And their progress was slow. An indication of this is that the family would usually end each year no more than 80 miles, as the crow flies, from where they had begun it. Though how many zigzagging miles had been covered in between, they alone knew. In Scotland, Katterfelto travelled somewhat faster, but even here he took six months to cover the 260 miles from Edinburgh, via Perth, Dundee and Aberdeen, to Inverness.

His progress was slow even by the standards of his own day. With the ever-expanding network of well-maintained toll-roads and the growing fleet of "Flying Machines" - as the horse-drawn coaches were sometimes grandly named - linking the major towns and cities, people could travel in a day the sort of distances that Katterfelto seemed to take months over. But then of course, with so much valuable equipment on board, his wagon probably went at no more than walking pace and Katterfelto was not going anywhere in particular. He was earning a living by working Britain in a systematic fashion. He was moving steadily between communities, usually staying in a local inn and performing, lecturing and exhibiting for anything between a few days to several months before he moved on.

This slow and thorough fifteen year coverage of much of Britain is in stark contrast to the frantic dash between the many European capitals that he claimed to have visited during the fifteen years before coming to Britain. Instead, perhaps we should visualise him moving at his slow, thorough pace through the towns and villages of just one or two European states. For the same reason, scepticism is appropriate over his claim to have visited Dublin.[30] The only period of time long enough to allow him to have made the journey would have been the four years before arriving in London in 1780.

However, the papers in the Irish capital at the time are strangely quiet on the subject. (Letters in the Dublin press during 1783 do in fact mention Katterfelto and show a detailed knowledge of his advertisements. However, the puffery they mock was very much 1783-style, when he was most definitely plying his trade in London. It seems that these letters simply show how far his fame had begun to spread.[31])

On at least three occasions Katterfelto's progress around Britain was made even slower than it already was by the intervention of the law. In 1805 an anonymous author wrote that, after having deceived London's population, Katterfelto

> *was not so successful in the provincial departments of the island; being often in danger of the stocks, and frequently obliged to make a precipitate retreat from the hands of justice, which, with all his knowledge and magic and divination, he could not always elude, for not long before his death, the Mayor of Shrewsbury committed him to the common House of Correction, as a vagrant and imposter!*[32]

It was, in fact, the autumn of 1793 and Katterfelto had made his way from Birmingham into Shropshire heading for Shrewsbury. He was also heading for trouble. Constables in the county were on a special look out for vagrants. That year they had been offered ten shillings a time for every one they apprehended. Human nature being what it is, it wasn't long before many of the constables realised that they could make a pretty profit by actually paying vagrants to come into their districts in order to be arrested.[33] Quite how much the vagrants received isn't clear, but it would need to have been enough to compensate them for the possible punishments they faced. While some were merely detained in the House of Correction and set to work there for a week, three months or even longer, others could be privately or publicly whipped. Still others were enrolled in the navy or "passed to the settlements" (in other words, deported). It seems that one day, in late 1793, a Constable may have come across a horse-drawn wagon driven by a strange foreign gentleman of the road and thought to himself: "It's payday!"

For Harry Houdini, Katterfelto was "a shining example of the social ostracism shown to show people"[34] but he was certainly not the first travelling entertainer to be imprisoned for plying his trade. Back in 1655 an order was made in Richmond, Yorkshire against constables for failing to apprehend "common players ... they being rogues by the statute",[35] while in 1684 the London Gazette carried an order suppressing "all mountebanks, rope-dancers and ballad-singers, who had not taken a licence from the Master of Revels."[36] These are just two of many attempts that were made over the years to regulate itinerant performers. By the time he arrived in Shrewsbury, Katterfelto had already fallen foul of these local by-laws elsewhere, as was announced in a parody of his adverts in the Cumberland Pacquet during 1790:

Wonders! On Wednesday last, the celebrated Doctor Katterfelto (M.D. and F.R.S.) was committed to the House of Correction at Kendal as a rogue and vagabond; and was also convicted of profane cursing and swearing, (very unseemly for a divine and moral philosopher) and paid the penalty inflicted by law for this offence. He had been previously informed by the magistrates, that he would not be permitted to perform his "juggling tricks" in the town, but placing too strong a reliance on the magic powers of his Morocco Black Cat, the Doctor disregarded the official warning, and so incurred the punishment and the disgrace. He has since been released, on making proper submission.[37]

His stay in the cells lasted just one night: not long enough for his temper to have cooled. He was not willing to let the matter lie. To Katterfelto, his imprisonment was "one of the most *surprising tricks* that ever was played in the whole world" and "the printers of the Cumberland Pacquet did very wrong in saying that the Doctor did *curse* and *swear*". Before departing "for London" to seek the aid of "the best Law",[38] he had one final message for the unappreciative people of the town. Knowing that there is only one thing worse than being talked about and that is not being talked about, he announced:

Doctor Katterfelto is a man of greatest eminence in England and it may now with truth be said that he is the topic of general conversation. He is by no means an admirer of the House of Correction at Kendal, though the building and its situation are commonly approved. He talks of "speaking to the King's Bench" on the subject of his night's residence at that place; on which some people affect to be witty, and observe that the Doctor (M.D. and F.R.S) has been so much

*accustomed to talking to empty benches, that he must be well
qualified to speak, even to the King's.* [39]

The details of the third, though earliest, of Katterfelto's brushes with
the law only emerged many years after his death. In 1831, with the
memory of the great man already beginning to fade, a letter was
published in a magazine called "The Mirror of Literature,
Amusement and Instruction" replying to the question: "Who was
Katerfelto?" (This misspelling of his name became commonplace.)
The writer had some wonderfully personal memories to share:

> *I became acquainted with him about the year 1790 or 1791,
> when he visited the City of Durham, accompanied by his wife
> and daughter. He then appeared to be about sixty years of age.
> His travelling equipage consisted of an old rumbling coach, a
> pair of sorry hacks, and two black servants. They wore green
> liveries with red collars, but the colours were sadly faded by
> long use.*
>
> *Having taken suitable apartments, the black servants
> were sent round the town, blowing trumpets and delivering
> bills, announcing their master's astonishing performances,
> which in the day time consisted in displaying the wonders of
> the microscope, &c. and in the evening in exhibiting electrical
> experiments, in the course of which he introduced his two
> celebrated black cats, generally denominated the Doctor's
> Devils—for, be it understood, that our hero went under the
> dignified style and title of Doctor Katerfelto. Tricks of
> legerdemain concluded the evening's entertainments.*
>
> *The first night of the Doctor's performance was extremely
> wet, and the writer of this, who was then quite a boy,
> composed his whole audience. The Doctor's spouse invited me
> behind the curtains to the fire, on one side of which sat the
> great conjuror himself, his person being enveloped in an old
> green, greasy roquelaire [a cloak], and his head decorated
> with a black velvet cap. On the other side of the fire-place sat
> Mrs. Katerfelto and daughter, in a corresponding style of
> dress—that is to say, equally ancient and uncleanly. The
> family appeared, indeed, to be in distressed circumstances.
> The Doctor told me the following odd anecdote: Some time
> before he had sent up from a town in Yorkshire a fire-
> balloon, for the amusement of the country people, and at*

which they were not a little astonished; but in a few days afterwards the Doctor was himself more astonished on being arrested for having set fire to a hay rick! The balloon, it appeared, had in its descent fallen upon a rick, which it consumed, and the owner, having ascertained by whom the combustible material had been dispatched, arrested the Doctor for the damage. As the Doctor was unable to pay the amount, he was obliged to go to prison, thus proving that it is sometimes easier to raise the devil than to "raise the wind." Having been admitted behind the scenes, I had an opportunity of seeing the conjuror's apparatus, but the performance was postponed to another evening.[40]

This memory from forty years before (Katterfelto actually visited Durham in 1787) gives us an intimate, behind the scenes picture of the man. So before we get carried away with thinking that he was a total rogue, spare a thought for him on that wet and dismal evening. He had attracted no audience and so had earned nothing to pay for the room or feed his family. And yet he had time to show this young lad his conjuror's apparatus and to tell a story in which he himself was the fall guy.

The letter also shows that just a few months after Thomas Montague had supposedly run away, Katterfelto was still making use of two black servants to drum (or rather trumpet) up business. We can also see that less than three years after leaving London the family had already fallen on hard times. The clothes in which the family performed were in a pretty poor state, while the faded uniforms of the servants seem in marked contrast to Thomas's smart and well-to-do outfit, with its white buttons, tassels, shoulder-knots and the like. The fine, strong horses remembered by Robert Hird in the previous decade were, by now, no more than "a pair of sorry hacks". As for hard cash, there wasn't enough to cover the value of a large pile of hay.

So much for the view of some of his detractors that Katterfelto was fleecing the nation by exploiting their gullibility. What he was actually trying to do was to make a living and provide for his family. He was simply "wondering for his bread", as the poet and hymn writer William Cowper had put it in "The Task" (possibly the most popular English poem of the latter part of the century). Yes, it served Katterfelto's purpose to talk up his earnings at times, and certainly to puff about how popular and successful his performances were -

after all, people aren't interested in seeing a flop. The reality though was quite different. The constant struggle that he had to attract the paying public to his shows can be seen from his ticket prices. The twenty-three years that Katterfelto toured the country saw prices for food and household items rise by 40%.[41] Despite this, the cost of seeing one his performances remained virtually unchanged: 2s 6d (or at most 3s) for the best seats, 2s for the middle seats and 1s for "servants and children" at the back.

As we shall see, the ever-enterprising Katterfelto responded to the economic challenges facing him by developing different exhibitions for which he could charge separately. He marketed a range of merchandise to supplement his income and, with times getting harder, he even took to bartering: offering tickets to the cutlery workers of Sheffield in return for some of their wares.[42] Most importantly of all, by regularly reinventing himself and presenting a variety of persona to the world, he broadened his appeal and managed the remarkable feat of surviving on the road, across Europe and in Britain, for some thirty-five years. Even so, as a travelling entertainer he would never earn a fortune. But fame? Now that was a different matter.

[1] See the shipping arrivals in the York Courant, 1st October 1766.
[2] No editions of the Hull Packet for September 1776 have survived.
[3] 26th-30th October 1787, The Edinburgh Advertiser
[4] Quoted in "The European Magazine and London Review", June 1783 (3), pages 406-9
[5] 5th June 1783, The General Advertiser, in Sophia Banks, A Collection of Broadsides, The British Library
[6] 10th August 1982, The Morning Post
[7] 16th April 1781, The Morning Post
[8] e.g. 15th July 1782, The Morning Post
[9] 29th November 1783, The General Advertiser, op cit
[10] 8th January 1785, The Norfolk Chronicle
[11] 6th June 1783, The General Advertiser, op cit
[12] The name could also be spelt Katterfeldt, Katterfeld, or Catterfeld
[13] 18th December 1784, The Norfolk Chronicle
[14] 29th October 1776, The York Courant
[15] The Conjuror's Repository, T and R Hughes, London, pages 92f
[16] Thomas Frost, The Lives of the Conjurors, 1786, chapter 6
[17] Theatre bill, 2nd February 1784, Whitby Museum
[18] Quoted in Modern Enchantments, Simon During, Harvard University Press,

2002, page 249

[19] The European Magazine, op cit

[20] Hird's Annals of Bedale, op cit, pages 218-221

[21] www.english-heritage.org.uk/server/show/nav.17488

[22] 24th November 1777, The Gloucester Journal

[23] 11th December 1780, The Morning Herald

[24] See the Journals of the House of Commons, 10th March 1773.

[25] The European Magazine, op cit

[26] 24th February 1786, The Lincoln, Rutland and Stamford Mercury

[27] 22nd January, 23rd February 1784, The Daily Advertiser, quoted in "Blake's London" by Paul Milner in "Studies in Romanticism", Volume 41, Issue 2, 2002, page 279f

[28] 29th June 1784, The General Advertiser, op cit

[29] 10th June 1784, The General Advertiser, op cit

[30] 8th January 1785, The Norfolk Chronicle (where he also claims to have visited Edinburgh); 25th April 1791, Williamson's Liverpool Advertiser

[31] Lyson's Collectanea Volume 1(2), pages 199f, dated "25th June 1783, Dublin G.P."

[32] Essay on Quackery and the Dreadful Consequences arising from taking Advertised Medicines, Anonymous, 1805, Kingston upon Hull, pages 62-3 (footnote)

[33] Records of the House of Quarter Session for the Co. of Salop, July 1801

[34] Houdini on Magic, ed. Walter Gibson and Morris Young, Dover Publications, 1953, page 57

[35] North Riding Quarter Sessions, Richmond, 12th January 1655

[36] Chambers Book of Days, Volume 1, 1888, entry for 14th April

[37] 12th May 1790, The Cumberland Pacquet

[38] 19th and 26th May 1790, The Cumberland Pacquet

[39] 2nd June 1790 The Cumberland Pacquet

[40] The Mirror of Literature, Amusement and Instruction; Volume 17, No.477, 19th February 1831

[41] Schumpeter-Gilbray Price Index in British Historical Facts 1760-1830, Chris Cook and John Stevenson, Macmillan, 1980

[42] 16th September 1796, The Iris or Sheffield Advertiser

CHAPTER 2

DR. BATTO AND HIS WORKS

"Katerfelto. A generic term for a quack or charlatan."
Brewer's Dictionary of Phrase and Fable, 1870

By the time Katterfelto left London in 1784 he had earned himself a reputation that was to last at least a hundred years. It was not exactly the reputation he had hoped for, but then for the showman no publicity is bad publicity. Almost exactly a century later, Dr. E. Cobham Brewer published his now much loved "Dictionary of Phrase and Fable". The entry for the word "Katerfelto" shows that, over the intervening decades, he had become so associated with quackery that his name had become synonymous with it. The story of how this came about takes us back into the world of eighteenth century medicine and to some of the most colourful characters of the time.

In the spring of 1782 influenza swept through the streets and houses of London. Especially among the poorer parts of the city, resistance to disease was already low. Here, among countless noisy street sellers, you could buy "fresh" water: fresh, that is, from the filthy Thames. Alternatively, you could drown your sorrows in one of the ubiquitous gin-houses, which were helping to lower fertility and bring on an early death. All this was contributing to some of the worst mortality rates in the capital since records began. (At one stage burials were exceeding baptisms by more than two to one.) So a new epidemic found easy access into people's lives and claimed many of them. For Katterfelto, ever the opportunist, it also proved to be a blessing in disguise. On the 15th April 1782 he announced to the world that

Mr KATTERFELTO is to exhibit the SOLAR MICROSCOPE, whereby he will shew those most

surprising insects, which have been advertised in the different papers, and have threatened this kingdom with a plague, if not speedily destroyed. They are the same kind, by all accounts, which caused a great plague in Italy in the year 1432.[1]

The flu epidemic continued through the month of June by which time it had claimed another victim:

Mr Katterfelto was taken very ill with the very alarming disorder that at present rages throughout this metropolis; the symptoms were a great weakness of the limbs, a swimming in the head, and a shivering of the whole body.

However, his good readers need not trouble themselves over his wellbeing because fortunately a helpful book was at hand:

He immediately had recourse to the celebrated Dr Batto's Works, and there found, that he had cured many thousand persons in Italy, in the year 1432, in the time of the plague. The air at that time in Italy was infected with a great number of insects as it is in the present here, besides those numerous insects which infect the hedges. At the time of Mr Katterfelto's being taken ill, he immediately tried the effect of Dr Batto's Medicines, and found himself perfectly recovered in 12 hours. Several persons have since been convinced of the amazing effect of this Medicine, and Mr Katterfelto as a Philosophic and Philanthropic, gives this public notice, that he has prepared a large quantity of the above invaluable Medicine, which will be sold (by him only) at the low price of Five Shillings the bottle, and will be signed and sealed by Mr Katterfelto.[2]

Since first going on sale four days earlier he claimed to have sold "above 200 bottles, which gained him great applause by the above Medicines".

Doubtless, the good Dr. Batto and his Works, containing the recipe for his medicine, are fictitious. There was certainly no known cure for the plague. Nor was there any way that "Dr. Batto" could have identified the "insects" (or microbes) responsible for it: for the simple reason that back in 1432 such things couldn't have been seen.

It wasn't until 1609 that Galileo first turned his lenses from the heavens to investigate the small things of the world. One of his students named the instrument a microscope, but it was a Dutchman, Anton van Leeuwenhoek, who in 1676 designed and made the more sophisticated microscopes with which he first saw and described the teeming organisms in a drop of water. (This achievement is also often attributed to the Englishman, Robert Hooke). Leeuwenhoek called these organisms "animalcules" and he found them everywhere, including on the plaque of his teeth and in faeces, though he did not associate them with disease.

Katterfelto's claim, that he had identified microscopic life forms as the cause of the flu epidemic, was unusual and controversial. In his day the predominant view was that most diseases were transmitted through "miasmas", or poisonous and foul smelling vapours. Katterfelto's view that illnesses such as plague were caused by miniature life forms had first been suggested by two fourteenth century Arabic scholars, Ibn Khatima and Ibn al-Khatib. It was then picked up in 1546 by an Italian, Girolamo Fracastoro, who proposed that the plague was transmitted by tiny "seminaria", or seeds. This idea of "contagion" gained a certain popularity but it wasn't until the nineteenth century that western medicine came to accept what we now call the germ theory of disease.

By siding with the theory of contagion Katterfelto was ahead of his time. He may even have believed that somewhere among his many types of "insect" there was one that really was responsible for the illness (although it wouldn't be until the 1930s that the flu virus would actually be identified). Not surprisingly, in his own day, many of his contemporaries had their doubts about his diagnosis for the flu. Despite this scepticism, Katterfelto reported that some in the medical establishment had demanded that the "insects" concerned be made available. This "request" provoked the following hostile response:

TREASONABLE CORRESPONDENCE
against the health of His Majesty's liege subjects

Whereas, besides the many important letters Dr Katterfelto has received, entreating his attendance in foreign Courts, he had last week divers epistles from Ireland, the Isles of Wight and Man, etc., etc., which he conceives to come from certain apothecaries, surgeons, and from others of the faculty, concerned in the destruction of the human race, as all those letters express a desire that he will set at liberty the dangerous insects now in his possession, and which occasioned the influenza last spring; which influenza the said writers seem desirous of having repeated, preferring their own emolument to the health of His Majesty's liege subjects, and for which purposes they offered Dr Katterfelto large sums of money in order to comply with their wishes.[3]

In contrast to such mercenary and irresponsible attitudes, the good doctor went on to reassure the public that the noxious insects would not be released again. However, they could be viewed quite safely through his microscope - at a price.

There was also much scepticism about the effectiveness of Dr. Batto's Medicine, despite the willingness of an anxious public to purchase it. According to the early nineteenth century "Essay on Quackery and the Dreadful Consequences arising from taking Advertised Medicines",

at this period a fellow, styling himself Dr Katterfelto, (who, besides a small smattering of medical jargon, had acquired the knowledge of a few sleight-of-hand tricks) advertised a nostrum, which he pronounced an infallible remedy for the prevailing malady; although it was clearly ascertained that the said nostrum consisted of nothing more than pure water, tinctured with some colouring ingredient, yet, so credulous were the public, that they eagerly sought after and purchased the non-effective trash.[4]

Reading this in an age of Complementary Medicine we are reminded of similar attacks made against the contents (or apparent lack of them) of homeopathic medicines. Homeopathy was, in fact, founded by a contemporary of Katterfelto and a fellow German, Samuel Hahnemann (1755-1843). However, we shouldn't imagine that Dr. Batto's "pure water" might actually be a homeopathic remedy. The first that Hahnemann published on the subject wasn't until 1796, fully fourteen years after the London epidemic.

Katterfelto's medical puffs brought him to the attention of many, including another German, Pastor Karl Philipp Moritz. In 1782 Moritz published his account of his travels around England in which he wrote of a certain gentleman who:

gives himself out for a Prussian, speaks bad English, and understands beside the usual electrical and philosophical experiments, some legerdemain tricks, with which (at least according to the papers) he sets the whole world in wonder. For in almost every newspaper that appears, there are some verses on the great Katterfelto, which some one or other of his hearers are said to have made extempore. Every sensible person considers Katterfelto as a puppy, an ignoramus, a braggadocio, and an impostor; notwithstanding which he has a number of followers. He has demonstrated to the people, that the influenza is occasioned by a small kind of insect, which poisons the air; and a nostrum, which he pretends to have found out to prevent or destroy it, is eagerly bought of him. A few days ago he put into the papers: "It is true that Mr. Katterfelto has always wished for cold and rainy weather, in order to destroy the pernicious insects in the air; but now, on the contrary, he wishes for nothing more than for fair weather, as his majesty and the whole royal family have determined, the first fine day, to be eye-witnesses of the great wonder, which this learned philosopher will render visible to them." Yet all this while the royal family have not so much as even thought of seeing the wonders of Mr. Katterfelto.[5]

By the summer of 1783 the flu was already long gone. Just in case it should return (and in the spring Katterfelto had spotted the insects "in the Air now again, but not so numerous"[6]) he let it be known that he still had a few bottles of Dr. Batto's to dispose of.[7] Otherwise, that was that - at least for the duration of his stay in London. Just a year's quackery, and yet such was the success of his self-publicity that by now Katterfelto's fame in this department was assured.

He was by no means the only quack to make use of newspapers in order to sell his wares. A small selection from them is sufficient to show that the needy yet discerning reader could avail him or herself of a whole variety of wonderful remedies. "Leake's justly famous Pill" promised to cure, in just fifteen days, such diverse ailments as venereal disease, scurvy and rheumatism. "A Cure for the bite of a mad dog" came with a testimony from the Vicar of Ormskirk, who seems to have faced considerable dangers during his parish visiting! The eighteenth century equivalent of Grecian 2000 for combating hair loss and grey hairs was, believe it or not, Bear Grease. Digestive problems could be tackled with the help of "Dr Wails Celebrated

Worm Medicine" in the form of gingerbread nuts. Should that fail then one could always turn to Worm Tea, which worked by "purging away such ropy and slimy Humours as are the Nests where these pernicious Vermin are bred in innumerable quantities." For those suffering from the even more intimate problem of incontinence, help was at hand in the shape (if that's quite the right word) of "Boogies of the Elastic Gum".

Nor was Katterfelto the only one to quote poetry in his own praise. Mr. Spilsbury, "Chemist", was able to call upon the services of one "Candidus" to support the efficacy of his product:

Blest be the Man, whose mental Powers impart
Health to the Body – Gladness to the Heart;
Whose friendly Hand hath op'd a ready Door
From complicated Ills to free the poor:
The SCURVY, fell Disease! no more appals
Abash'd – dismay'd – the Hydra Monster falls
No more to rise, - He yields the dubious Day,
And with reluctance quits his destin'd Prey.[8]

The "hydra monster" of scurvy, slain by Mr. Spilsbury, was a major threat to life in the Navy. At the time there was no cure for it while at sea, although it was known that once on shore sufferers stood a good chance of recovering by eating such things as wild celery, wood sorrel and nasturtiums. However, there was also a superstition among sailors that touching or smelling the earth was the best cure. This led a Danish navigator, by the name of Vitus Bering, to have himself half buried in the ground in the hope of a cure - a vain hope as it turned out, but it may have lessened the work involved at his funeral! As well as scurvy, the good Mr. Spilsbury offered to cure such illnesses as gout, leprosy and "King's Evil". The "Evil", or scrofula, was an often-fatal inflammation of the lymph glands in the neck. It gained its name from the belief that it could only be healed by the touch of a king or queen, until, that is, Mr. Spilsbury came along.

There seems to have been a remarkable lack of squeamishness about what the eighteenth century reader could be faced with at the breakfast table, with front page adverts for the treatment of gonorrhoea - opium was one recommended cure. Nor did the medical salesmen shun away from problems of the inner self. "Dr Henry's Chemical Nervous Medicine" never failed to give relief from all nervous complaints, such as:

hypochondriac melancholy, hysteric vapours, langours, palpitations and trembling of the heart, giddiness, violent head-achs, noise in the ears, mists before the eyes, swimming in the head, fainting, lowness of spirits, obstructions in the capillary vessels, weakness of the brain, flushing in the face, irregular thoughts, agitation in the stomach and bowels; in short, all disorders proceeding from wind and indigestion.[9]

Many of the medicines were heavily marketed and distributed wholesale, such as Hooper's Female Pills and Dr. James's Fever Powders. The profits could be enormous and Mr. Hooper found it necessary to defend his source of income by cautioning his customers against counterfeit versions of his pills.[10] Another person to do well was Nathaniel Gobold, a baker who earned around £10,000 a year from sales of his Vegetable Balsam. However, it was not only the quacks who benefited from the publicity that the newspapers made possible. The papers themselves depended heavily on the advertising revenues brought in by these practitioners. In fact, the newspaper proprietors sometimes acted as sales outlets, distributing the medicines. For example the Leeds Messenger in the 1790s was printed by Thomas Wright, who respectfully informed "the inhabitants of Leeds and the places adjacent that he has just received a fresh supply of Medicines from Manchester."[11] (The medicines concerned were "Lignums Antiscorbatic Drops" - good for leprosy, scurvy and scrophula.)

The media-savvy Georgian quack had clearly come a long way since the one-man band of the Tudor and Stuart "mountebank". These were so called because they mounted benches (or "banks") in order to hold forth to the crowds at fairs and in market places. Back then, the language used was even choicer than in Katterfelto's days. Ben Johnson, the Elizabethan playwright, had offered a wonderful definition of a quack as "a turdy-facy-nasty-paty-fartical rogue". Even better was the seventeenth century mountebank who offered to cure the conditions gloriously referred to as "the Glimmering of the Gizzard, the Quivering of the Kidneys, and the Wambling Trot."[12] (Try those on your Doctor at your next visit!) In the early part of the eighteenth century, mountebanks were still numbered among the travelling showmen. They regularly gave themselves spurious biographical details and various airs and graces, as one traveller through England recounted in 1723:

I cannot leave Winchester without telling you of a pleasant incident that happened there. As I sat at the George Inn, I saw a coach with six bay horses, a calash and four, and a chaise and four, enter the inn in a yellow livery turned up with red; four gentlemen on horseback, in blue trimmed with silver; and as yellow is the colour given by the dukes in England, I went out to see what duke it was. ... Upon enquiry I found this great equipage belonged to a mountebank. ... The footmen in yellow were his tumblers and trumpeters, and those in blue his merry-andrew [a jester], his apothecary and spokesman. He was dressed in black velvet and had in his coach a woman that danced on the ropes. He cures all diseases and sells his packets for sixpence-a-piece. He erected stages in all the market towns twenty miles around; and it is a prodigy how so wise a people as the English are gulled by such pick-pockets.[13]

By the late eighteenth century these flamboyant quacks had become, in large part, more businessmen than showmen, although many still travelled the country. Using new entrepreneurial skills and the ever-expanding circulation of newspapers, they were able to make their sales pitches to a much wider audience of a fashionable elite with a growing disposable income.

Many medical "irregulars" were in fact well intentioned and quite skilful, or at least as skilful as the medical establishment, though this isn't necessarily saying that much. One leading physic, Dr. Radcliffe, was prepared to admit that most medicine and therapy on offer by regular medics was actually useless. Many of the cures supplied by eighteenth century medicine relied quite heavily on the placebo effect, although some did include ingredients that really worked. Opium brought relief from pain and congestion, as well as acting as a sedative, and mercury was effective in treating venereal disease, although both ingredients could have some fairly serious side effects of their own. Fevers could be brought down with the help of antimony, while rhubarb, aloes, and senna were useful in purging the bowels. However, there was an array of illnesses, whether life threatening or "merely" disabling, disfiguring or painful, for which there was no established remedy.

The lack of effective cures for most illnesses led the general population to pick and mix between regular and irregular approaches. Many would try anything in the quite understandable desire to get well. Medical practitioners of all kinds sprang up everywhere and in one way or another sought to make a living in a society rife with ill health. As for "quackery", whatever it was, it was always something that someone else did. The desire of irregular practitioners to distance themselves from their rivals, and not to be labelled as quacks themselves, is illustrated in the announcement of the following publication by the scurvy-slaying Mr. Spilsbury:

> *Free Thoughts on Quacks and their Medicines occasioned by the death of Dr Goldsmith and Mr Scawen, or a candid and ingenious inquiry into the Merits and Dangers imputed to advertised Remedies. Dedicated to both Houses of Parliament. By F.Spilsbury Chemist – seller of his justly celebrated Anti-Ascorbic Drops.[14]*

The commercialisation of, and competition within, the medicine trade was a sign that Britain was becoming a consumer society. There were many who had spare money in their pockets and fashionable practitioners could hope to part them from it. Katterfelto was admirably placed to cash in. He had all the mountebank skills of the showman and, as we have seen, he copied their practice of creating elaborate and fictitious biographies. Above all, he was the supreme exponent of promoting himself through the media. Yet for all his bluster about how much he earned, it was others who made their fortunes from the quack medicine trade. For Katterfelto it was fame rather than fortune that came his way. This fame was stimulated not only by his own advertisements but also by those who began to satirise him.

On the 17th March 1783 a cartoon was published called "The Quacks". It was based on a rivalry that had developed between Katterfelto and Doctor James Graham, another exotic character of the time. In the picture, the two men are facing up against each other like generals in battle. Cannons pointing across the divide, and the skull and cross bones insignia of the Death's Head Hussars, both serve to emphasise the mock-military setting. Katterfelto appears among some of the electrical paraphernalia from his shows, with his hair standing on end as if charged by static, and with electricity spouting from his thumb and forefinger. In broken and heavily accented English he issues a gladiatorial challenge to his opponent:

> *Dare you was see de Vonders of the Vorld, which make de hair Stand on tiptoe. Dare you was see mine Tumb and mine findgar, Fire from mine findgar and Feaders on mine Tumb –*

1. The Quacks

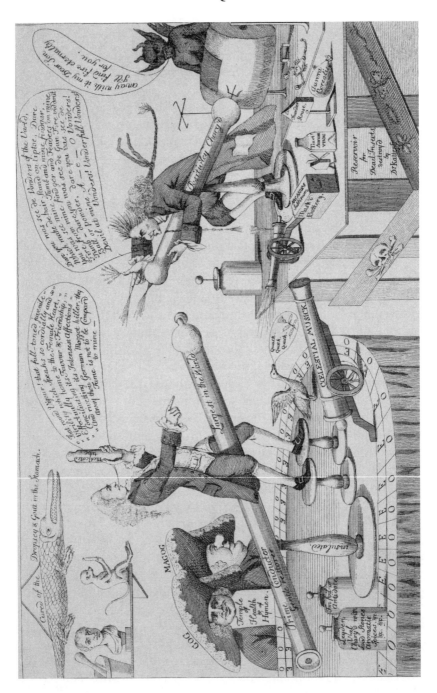

dare you was see de Gun Fire viddout Ball or powder, dare
you was see de Devil at mine A— e
– O Vonders! Vonders! Vonderful Vonders!

At his rear, or his "A— e", as the cartoon delicately puts it, stands a
female demon who declares: "Away with it my Dear Son, I'll find
fire eternally for you."

The cartoon satirises many aspects of Katterfelto's performances,
such as the way he mingled scientific lectures with entertainment and
suggestions that he was in touch with the "dark side". His
microscopic wonders are portrayed in literal fashion as a butterfly,
centipede, moth and worm in a "Reservoir for Dead Insects
destroyed by Dr Katterfelto". It also mocks his style of delivery and
command of the language, while his patched frock coat indicates,
either that he was not as well off as he claimed, or that he preferred
to spend his money on such things as equipment for his shows.

What is surprising is that, in a cartoon called "The Quacks", there
is only one explicit reference to his forays into the world of medicine.
This is the little bottle labelled "Tinct^r Aurum Vivae", i.e. "Tincture
of the gold of living [water?]". (This may be an allusion to the elixir,
the philosopher's stone, which, as well as turning base metals to gold,
was also believed to cure all ills and prolong life indefinitely.) The
static electricity illustrated in the cartoon also had strong medical
connotations by his time. However, although Katterfelto used it in
various ways in his lecture-shows to amaze his audiences, he doesn't
appear to have tapped into its medical potential until almost a decade
later, as we shall see. Clearly there was much about Katterfelto to
make fun of. Yet just as clearly he was going to be remembered in
large part as a quack, even if, as the cartoon itself shows, this was only
a small aspect of what he was about.

By the 1780s static electricity was being widely used in medical
circles and was one of the modern wonders of the world. More and
more people became convinced of the healing power of "Medical
Electricity" and the ailments that succumbed to it were supposedly
legion. One early advocate had been John Wesley, the founder of
Methodism. Wesley believed that established medicine was a
conspiracy of the professionals against the laity and that a person
was more likely to die in hospital than out of it. So he set up free
medical clinics for the poor of Bristol and London, and introduced
electrical machines into them to serve the masses. In 1756, his
Journal records his views on "the virtue of this surprising

medicine", expressing his conviction that "to this day, while hundreds, perhaps thousands, have received unspeakable good, I have not known one man, woman, or child, who has received hurt thereby."[15]

However, accounts of healings by Wesley's lower class of patient were given little credibility in a culture where only the testimony of a "gentleman" was thought to be reliable. Being new and experimental it was perhaps inevitable that some would regard the "electrifying" of patients as quackery, irrespective of whether or not it was effective. Typical of the criticisms levelled at exponents of this approach was a poem entitled "On the raging Taste for ELECTRICITY" submitted to Felix Farley's Bristol Journal:

Some Virtuous – not for gain,
(With bottle – wire – tube – and chain)
Persuade the credulous to try
to ease the pain of leg or thigh;
Or if a finger, or a toe,
Their grand machine will cure the woe.
This plaything, now is twirled around,
By men of wealth, to cobblers down –
Too many with simplicity,
Put faith in electricity,
Tho' 'tis observed by young and old,
It never yet has cured a cold
Nor any pain – but makes it fly,
from head to foot – from hand to eye,
As Quacks in managing the gout
Divert the pain – not drive it out. ....
The famous Ward – (if not bely'd)
His Pill and Drop, on puppies try'd,
Then practis'd on the very poor,
And gratis strove to ease or cure,
But when his Medicines were known
They sunk in fame – fell lowly down.
So will it fare with tube and wire
When folks are sick of shock and fire.[16]

One who shared more than most in this fever of medical electrical activity was Katterfelto's rival in the "Quacks" cartoon, Dr. Graham. James Graham was another highly colourful character in the ranks of late eighteenth century eccentricity and one of the most famous and fashionable medical irregulars of the period.

By the time Katterfelto was making his first visit to York in 1776, Graham, who had studied medicine in Edinburgh, was practising in London and Bath and was already showing symptoms of what the regular practitioners would have diagnosed as a case of full-blown quackery. He was curing a vast range of ailments by therapies that included diet, magnetism, baths and vapours.[17] He had also begun to make extensive use of large and highly decorated pieces of "medico-electrical apparatus." Graham became very popular in the fashionable circles of Bath, but what really brought him to the attention of the nation were his lectures in London, which were the Georgian equivalent of "The Joy of Sex".

He began to deliver these in the autumn of 1779 in his exotically named "Temple of Health and Hymen" situated in the Adelphi Buildings on the riverside near the Strand (and later in Pall Mall). The Temple was elaborately decorated and the suitability of the clientele was preserved by two enormous footmen (pictured as Gog and Magog in the "Quacks" cartoon). The centrepiece of the Temple was without doubt his famous Celestial Bed. By all accounts it was quite a sight. Twelve feet long and nine feet wide, the bed was covered in pink sheets and supported by forty glass pillars. It was covered with a dome lined with mirrors and was engraved with the words "Be fruitful and multiply and replenish the earth". The motto pointed to its purpose: wealthy but childless couples could hire the bed, at the rate of fifty pounds per night, in order to cure their infertility. This was to be brought about with the help of the vast magnets and electrical machines that were attached to the bed. How many takers there were is not recorded, nor how fruitful the result.

In addition to exhibiting grand and risqué furniture Dr. Graham lectured on topics that were equally risqué:

He will give a curious and very eccentric lecture on the propagation of the human species and on the means of exalting and rendering permanent the joys of the Marriage Bed, producing a numerous, healthy and beautiful offspring, and of preserving even to a good old age, that round permanent vigour, that full-toned juvenile virility, which are so necessary to the honour and happiness of the individual, as well as to the strength and prosperity of the State; and which, moreover, speaks so cordially and so effectually home to the female heart.[18]

Not surprisingly this caused something of a stir. Some of these phrases were quoted in the "Quacks" cartoon, which satirised Graham as "Doctor Sex", seating him upon a phallic tube on which is written: "Largest in the World". Graham regularly complained about the widespread prejudice against the Temple, the celestial bed and his lectures. To try to counter this, readers of the London papers were repeatedly informed that

> *The Ladies and Gentlemen who honour Dr Graham with their company, may be assured that everything will be conducted with the decency and decorum which cannot fail to establish the credit of this most useful institution, and silence effectually ignorant, envious or malevolent tongues.*[19]

Despite these assurances Graham was soon advertising a lecture "calculated for GENTLEMEN". These "men only" audiences heard that part of the secret of a long and healthy life lay in energetic sexual performance. They learnt that the use of erotica, which was quite prevalent in Georgian times, could be an aid to sex. They were even told that wives could learn valuable lessons in the erotic arts from prostitutes, although prostitution itself, like masturbation, was a depraved practice. No doubt they were also suitably entertained by the diaphanously clad young ladies who posed as nymphs in the Temple. One of these was, reputedly, the society beauty Emma Lyons who later became Lady Hamilton, the mistress of Admiral Lord Nelson.

Ladies were also catered for with lectures of their own. These were delivered by the High Priestess of the Temple, "Vestina Gigantica", or "the rosy, the gigantick, the stupendous Goddess of Health",[20] who sat upon her "Celestial Throne" instructing the ladies in "the Causes, Nature and Effect of Love and Beauty". Despite Graham's assurances that "the most strictly virtuous lady in the world, or even Virgin-Angels themselves, may be present at the whole lecture",[21] it is not surprising that some ladies preferred to go to the Temple incognito. This led Graham to appeal to the Magistrate to allow the wearing of masks at the Temple, only to be told that the practice was "in no way legal".[22]

This was not the end of the Magistrate's interest in the goings-on at Doctor Graham's establishment. In the "Quacks" cartoon, the table on which Graham and his equipment are set is an E.O. table. E.O. was a popular but illegal gambling game, which could be played at the Temple of Health. On the 29th July 1782 the Temple was raided and several tables were cut up. Three days later another raid took place and two more tables were broken, as was the head of one of the Justices who was severely hurt in the uproar. Six men were later prosecuted "for keeping a Common Gaming House for playing at E.O. at Dr. Graham's in Pall Mall", and the crime was compounded when someone attempted to bribe some of the witnesses for the prosecution to change their evidence.[23] Dr. Graham responded in the press to this public relations disaster by rejecting the reports made by "envious and malevolent persons" that he was benefiting from the gaming tables in his apartments.[24]

One of these "persons" was Katterfelto who had begun taking swipes at E.O. in his adverts earlier in the month. Shortly after the raids on Graham's establishment Katterfelto exploited his rival's woes even further:

Destructive E.O., fashionable sport,
To which, in crowds, th'unthinking world resort;
By you expos'd, appears in proper view,
And bids you shun what may in time undo.[25]

The "Quacks" cartoon suggests that Graham hit back, calling Katterfelto the "German Maggot Killer".

Doctor Graham's lectures went far beyond advice on sex. He also explained how the population of Great Britain could be not only doubled but made "infinitely more brilliant and vigorous."[26] Not only was the Celestial Bed able to increase fertility, it could also enhance the quality of the offspring conceived upon it. Its widespread use would lead to

the propagation of Beings rational and far stronger and more
beautiful in mental as well as bodily endowments than the
present puny, feeble, and nonsensical race of Christians, of
probationary immortals, who crawl and fret, and, contrary to
every principle of reason, humanity, national policy, and of
Christianity, persecute, rob, destroy and cut one another's
throats for nothing at all on most parts of this Terrageous
globe.[27]

The potential impact he had in mind was illustrated by the following contrast, one that now seems in very bad taste:

The Rosy Herald of Health, of the most gigantic stature that ever was seen in England, being between seven and eight feet high and a Dwarf lady will exhibit striking specimens; the former of the strength and stature of that race of beings which would spring from the Celestial Bed, and the latter of the present puny degeneration of mankind, which a due attention to the precepts inculcated in that Lecture would effectually improve.[28]

Not only would following the doctor's prescriptions enhance the quality of the human stock, it would also prolong human life to as yet unimagined lengths. In 1783 Graham offered a free lecture on "the simplest, most rational, and most certain means, in regard of air, exercise, eating, drinking, and other communications (without medicines) of preserving life healthily, happily, usefully and honourably, till at least an hundred and fifty years of age".[29]

One of the more unusual aspects of Graham's life-prolonging approach to medicine was earth-bathing. The healing properties of the soil have been attested to by many a gardener. They had also been tried, but found wanting, by Vitus Bering in his search for a cure for scurvy. However, whereas the Danish navigator had only been buried up to the waist, Dr. Graham went much further, being immersed right up to his lips. In doing so he claimed to have found a remedy that was good for more, much more, than just scurvy. He discovered,

with astonishment and delight, that planting the naked body long and repeatedly in the earth, most naturally, safely, speedily and effectually cures the foulest, most malignant, and most fatal species and degrees of the Sea and Land Scurvy, asthmatic, consumptive, serophulous, rheumatic, leprous, venereal, dropsical, cancerous, paralytic and nervous diseases; white and other swellings, insanity, the worst fevers, and all internal and external pains, inflammations, itchings and ulcers; or, in a word, that Earth-Bathing most effectually cleanses the human body and limbs from all impurities, abstracts from them every species and degree of poison and diseasedness, even those occasioned by the bite of mad animals, and saturates or charges them with the greatest measure of freshness, sweetness, strength and alacrity, which the constitution of the individual is capable.[30]

According to Graham, earth-bathing was, potentially, of more benefit than "all the Surgeons, Apothecaries, Physicians, Hospitals and Infirmaries", because it was impossible for any disease to continue when someone is "planted naked again in the womb of the all-fostering bosom of our original mother – the sweet, mellow, fresh, living, and life and strength-giving earth".[31]

As one eyewitness recalled, the problem of how to be buried naked in a hole in the ground in full view of the public was solved in the following fashion:

After making his bow he seated himself on the stool; when two men with shovels began to place mould in the cavity; as it approached to the pit of the stomach he kept lifting up his shirt, and at last he took it entirely off, the earth being up to his chin, and the doctor being left in puris naturalibus. He then began his lecture, expatiating on the excellent qualities of the Earth Bath, how invigorating etc - quite enough to call up the chaste blushes of the modest ladies.[32]

If all this wasn't enough to convince (or scandalise) the crowds, then Graham threw in the prospect of seeing not only himself being buried naked but also his young lady companion. As an onlooker reported, she "had her hair elaborately dressed in the prevailing fashion, with powder, flowers, feathers and ropes of pearl; the doctor appearing in an equally elaborate wig." Once buried, with just their powdered faces and wigs above ground, they looked "not unlike two fine, full-grown cauliflowers".[33] Graham maintained this position for up to six hours and claimed to have repeated it some two hundred times.[34]

The final years of Graham's life were spent in Edinburgh where his increasing eccentricity appears to have tipped over into actual mental instability or illness. One witness wrote of how the doctor would "madden himself with opium, rush out into the streets, and strip himself to clothe the first beggar he met";[35] he was also confined for a time as a lunatic. In a tract published in 1793 he testified that for sixteen days he had eaten and drunk nothing except water, had worn only cut up turfs against his skin, and had rubbed his limbs with his own nervous "aethereal balsam". The tract was subtitled "How to live for many weeks, months or years without eating anything whatever." He died the following year: sadly not at the ripe old age of one hundred and fifty as he had hoped, but just forty-nine.

Despite their earlier rivalry, or perhaps because of it, Katterfelto and Graham had found themselves appearing together not only in prints such as "The Quacks" but also in song. "The West Country Puffing Family" was a popular ditty celebrating their skills in boastful self-aggrandisement. It was "dedicated to those Princes of Puffs who exist at their Wholesale Puff-a-de-Puff Wharehouses, the Sign of the Devil and Black Cat, Piccadilly; and the Temple of Health, Pall Mall." The last verse ran:

> *Thus Puffing's become now the Trade,*
> *Of Katterfelto and Graham well known,*
> *Whose mouths confessedly are made,*
> *For nought else but Puffing alone.*[36]

It can't be denied that the two doctors were the unsurpassed masters of the art. They were certainly major contributors to what one commentator saw as "the monstrous and unprecedented height to which the arts of *puffing* … [have] arrived at in this town; by which the vilest and most contemptible productions are extolled".[37] No doubt this made them fair game. However, while James Graham was a thoroughgoing, if highly irregular, medical practitioner, Katterfelto was more of a dabbler in the art.

This becomes clear after Katterfelto leaves London to resume his travels. Despite the success of Dr. Batto's works and the publicity surrounding them, it would be a full four years before he showed any sign of playing the quack card once again. By then he had begun to find making a living increasingly hard, and following his visit to Edinburgh, the medical capital of Scotland, it seems to have occurred to him that one more way to supplement his income would be if he developed his medical credentials. So, by the time he reached Aberdeen in the summer of 1788 he had begun to adopt a new style of address: "Dr Katterfelto MD".[38] He had been using the title of Doctor for at least five years, but until now he had only ever been claiming to be a Doctor of Philosophy, never of Medicine.

Outrageous as Katterfelto's glib assumption of a medical qualification may seem to us, there was nothing in the society of the time to prevent him from doing so. The top tier of the medical establishment was indeed made up of university-trained "physicians". Yet outside of London there was no regulatory or licensing system and so there were no penalties for those who made unwarranted claims to be "Gentlemen of the Faculty". (How different this was from the situation in Germany from where Hahnemann and his Homeopathy were drummed out.)

Now though, with his medical credentials established, Katterfelto was in a position to offer Georgian society the benefit of his skills and experience. In July 1789 the people of Glasgow woke up to read in their morning paper that

Dr Katterfelto is very glad it has been in his power, during these four weeks past, to cure several persons of hardness of hearing, rheumatic, ague, and paralytic disorders, and such as have weak eyes and green wounds.[39]

From now on quackery would be a regular, though by no means constant feature of his publicity. By the time he arrived at Birmingham in 1792 he was claiming to cure complaints that many other doctors would not touch.[40] He had also joined the national grid of electrical healers, electrifying for free those who had various complaints.[41] He went on to explain, as a

Master of all the wonder-working art,
Of separate elements, with varied force,
How fire electric, swiftly thro' each part
With healing aid pursues its subtle course.[42]

He claimed some success in relieving "Nervous Disorders"[43] and often expressed the hope that "the blind and lame would try his skill".[44] He also frequently offered people two tinctures for sale: not the "Aurum Vivae" of the "Quacks" cartoon but one "for curing the Tooth-Ach in five Minutes"[45] and another "most valuable Tincture for the Cure of violent Head-Achs, Sprains, Bruises and Rheumatic Pains, which never fails of curing."[46] (This latter pain-reliever was advertised for sale at Shrewsbury and was perhaps another reason for the Mayor of that town to imprison him as an impostor!)

Over time, Katterfelto M.D. was able to claim in various places that "The different capital CURES he has performed in this town since his arrival would fill a whole news-paper." [47] However, lest people should think that he was just another medical con-artist he would regularly add: "His Plea is, - no Cure, no Pay."[48] Not only that but, in keeping with the charitable tendencies of other travelling healers such as Dr. Graham, he was often able to perform "several very capital cures (gratis) on the poor."[49] Those who did have to pay would be pleased to find that it was all done on "on very low terms."[50] Despite this, on leaving Birmingham he was forced to remind people, who were "indebted to him according to promise of Payment", to cough up for their cure and not to give him "any further Trouble".[51]

One new therapy that Katterfelto occasionally flirted with was the brainchild of the German physician Franz Mesmer. Mesmer claimed that "magnetic fluid" was present in all living beings and that if its flow was interrupted then all sorts of ailments followed. Outwardly, Mesmer's treatments, which he called "animal magnetism", involved such things as making passes with his hands down the arms of his patients; pressing below their diaphragm for anything up to three hours; and, in a precursor of hypnotism, staring intently into the patient's eyes so as to create a therapeutic bond. Inwardly, the effect of all this was, Mesmer claimed, to rebalance the flow of magnetic fluid, thus restoring the patient to health.

"Animal magnetism" caused quite a stir. People were cured but ladies swooned at Mesmer's touch and indecent rumours spread. He fled from Vienna to Paris but scandal followed close behind. A Royal Commission was set up by Louis XVI, which found no evidence for the existence of any such magnetic fluid. It concluded that, whatever the benefits of Mesmer's treatments might be, they were due to "imagination". Franz Mesmer was driven into exile soon after.

In Britain, this new therapy (sometimes later known as "mesmerism") did not attract many followers. As The Times put it in 1790: "To the honour of this country, the weak people that are influenced by the folly of Animal Magnetism are but few."[52] Several highly expensive practitioners did set up in London and elsewhere, stimulating public debates on the subject, such as: "Are the cures attributed to Animal Magnetism performed by the operation of conceit in the patients, the power of Satanic influence, some occult principles in philosophy, or is the whole an imposition of interested persons to take advantage of the credulity of Mankind."[53] Others were not slow to exploit the possible *double entrendre* in the name of this new medical treatment, such as one who lampooned Katterfelto and Graham in the process:

Among the wonders of this present most wonderful age, nothing can be so wonderful and surprising, (since the most renowned, most surprising, most wonderful Doctor Katterfelto and his Black Cat) as is now offered to the public by the Animal Doctor, who instead of a Black Cat, produces a much more wonderful, intelligent and animated Animal – a

great Jack Ass, whose powers, by the effects of the Doctor's
animal magnetism, surpasses even Graham's electrical bed so
much talked of for some time since, by all ladies of high
breeding ... He undertakes to perfect, in this most wonderful
act of producing animal magnetism, all disappointed misses,
wives, and forsaken widows, for the moderate sum of 50
pounds each, or ten pounds per month attendance at his
lectures. This wonderful Doctor assures the public, it is with
concern he is obliged to defer taking more than two patients
at a time in his house; from the great call he has of late had,
rendering him incapable to do justice to more at a time at
present. He begs the ladies who do him the honour to attend
his lectures, to be so good as to believe the effect of his animal
magnetism is, for the sake of decency, better imagined than
described.
    signed An Englishman[54]

Nevertheless, throughout the 1790s Katterfelto judged that there was
sufficient interest in the subject to include it in his lectures. At
Chester in 1791 he began to explain the principles of animal
magnetism as it was being "delivered at Bath" (probably by Dr.
Mainauduc who was practising around this time in Bristol) and in
London by a John Holloway. In deliberate contrast to their
supposed charges (three guineas and five guineas a time) Katterfelto
offered to explain it "gratis".[55] Over the next few years he continued
to demonstrate and lecture about animal magnetism.[56] However, he
also made the most of its multiple meanings to illustrate the allure of
his feline friend and his own magnetic personality:

    The Doctor's levee indeed yesterday was crowded, in short his
    cat again seems to possess a sort of animal magnetism and
    himself like his loadstone is all attraction![57]

For all Katterfelto's dabbling in the applied side of quackery, he
never lost sight of his higher aim of not simply curing the sick but
enabling the healthy to remain so. He did this by opening up to them
a new world of understanding. Audiences in Whitehaven witnessed
"various useful and wonderful experiments in the Medical line".[58]
Likewise, with the help of his solar microscope the people of Chester
were introduced to
    the effects of arsenic and mercury sublimate, how they operate

on the person, also the real goodness and badness of a person's blood, also the effects of medicine, and how to escape various disorders and diseases; likewise the badness of some lancets, [surgical knives used, for example, in blood-letting] which often prove dangerous to ladies and gentlemen and how to prevent a person from having the tooth-ach.[59]

Katterfelto was not the only person to be aware of the dangers of mercury, which was used to treat venereal disease. For example Dr. Wheatley's Remedies for the Itch were sold "by the King's Authority" and promised relief within four hours without the aid of mercury. However, the advantage that his microscope gave Katterfelto over other practitioners was the ability to extend medical understanding by showing "the real cause, whence different disorders and diseases arise".[60] The most obvious example of this was, of course, that

he did discover seven years ago in London, the real Cause of the Influenza, and likewise at that time did cure many of the very first Nobility of that violent Disorder, which was the Cause he became a Favourite of the Majesties.[61]

Katterfelto's purported medical relationship with the royals had not ended when he left London. In 1789 he wrote that

He is also glad that his Three Letters of Advice, which he sent to the Queen and Prince of Wales, above Twelve Months ago, did also prove a great Benefit to the King's Health.[62]

This concern for the health of King George III, shared by most of the nation, was at a time when the King was suffering from his first period of what seemed to be mental illness. This manifested itself in bouts of agitation and continual ranting that were so severe that he had to be restrained in a straitjacket and chained to a chair. The King did recover through the unorthodox but humane psychiatric methods of Dr. Francis Willis. However, the illness returned at the start of the next century and in 1810 he went blind and became permanently incapable of carrying out his royal duties. The following year Parliament passed the Regency Bill and appointed his eldest son to rule as Prince Regent until the King's death in 1820.

Katterfelto was not the only practitioner to send advice to the

Royal Family about their health. In 1791, his rival Doctor Graham announced to the public of Liverpool that he had written to the Prince of Wales, saying that the heir to the throne would suffer from the same affliction as his father if he did not marry a certain princess. (By this he meant that the Prince needed to embrace Evangelical Christianity, to which Graham had been converted two years earlier).[63]

Despite Graham's conviction, the King's condition was not a punishment sent from God. In the 1970s, "the madness of King George" was finally diagnosed as a very severe case of a blood condition known as porphyria. That this, in turn, had been triggered by arsenic poisoning was revealed in 2004, when analyses of samples of the king's hair showed that it contained three hundred times more than the safe level of the chemical. This extraordinary amount was partly the result of a steady build-up over many years of the arsenic contained in his skin cream and wig-powder. However, the key discovery was that when he was suffering from his fits the King was given Dr. James's Fever Powders (mentioned above) several times a day. These powders were made of antimony, and antimony contains significant amounts of arsenic. So the very medication he was being given for his illness was only serving to poison him more and make the attacks even worse.[64]

If this had been known at the time it would certainly have been bad news for Dr. James. Yet it could hardly have made some of the attacks on irregular medicine any more virulent than they already were. For example, one of quackery's cultured despisers accused its practitioners of being a "race of destroyers" who were "in the continual habit of sending myriads to an untimely grave."[65] Given this level of hostility between some in the medical establishment and the irregulars, it was probably a vain, though oft-repeated, hope of Katterfelto's that "the Gentlemen of the Faculty" would come from far and wide to see his wonders, medical and otherwise.[66]

Katterfelto certainly suffered from a serious case of quackery. The first onset came during the flu epidemic in London and there were continual recurrences throughout the last ten years of his life. In some ways he was a throwback to the earlier days of the mountebank with his showmanship and fake biography. Yet, in his later years, tinctures and treatments only featured at the end of his advertisements. What always came first was his more elevated aim of extending public understanding of the mysteries of the universe. His quackery might all have been a fiddle - but for him it always played second fiddle. This is somewhat ironic given that, with his countless rivals, many of whom were far more successful than him, it was his name alone that became synonymous with quackery. But then that is a testimony to the extraordinary effect of his puffs during his time in London. While the medical trade added another string to his bow, and was a source of income that he could not afford to overlook, it was certainly not the main part of Katterfelto's self-image or public persona. He was determined not to be confused with the common-or-garden quack. Rather his mind was set upon higher things.

[1] 15th April 1782, The Morning Herald

[2] 3rd June 1782, The General Advertiser, op cit

[3] Quoted in "Houdini on Magic", op cit, page 63

[4] Essay on Quackery, op cit

[5] Travels in England in 1782, Karl Philipp Moritz, 1886, Cassell, pages 70-71

[6] 2nd April 1783, The Daily Advertiser

[7] 26th August 1783, The Morning Post

[8] 8th October 1776, The York Courant

[9] 25th October 1776, The York Chronicle

[10] The Newcastle Courant during April 1787

[11] 30th July 1798, The Leeds Messenger

[12] Roy Porter, "Before the Fringe: Quack Medicine in Georgian England", History Today, Volume 36, Issue 11, November 1986, pages 16-22. In this chapter I am indebted to Roy Porter's work, especially "Quacks", Tempus, 2000.

[13] Chambers Book of Days, op cit

[14] 8th May 1777, Felix Farley's Bristol Journal

[15] John Wesley, The Journal of the Rev John Wesley, 9th November 1756

[16] 16th March 1778, Felix Farley's Bristol Journal

[17] 1st May 1777, Felix Farley's Bristol Journal

[18] 24th July 1782, The Morning Post

[19] 10th July 1781, The Morning Post

[20] 25th March 1783, The Daily Advertiser

[21] 5th December 1783, The Morning Post

[22] 9th May 1782, The London Courant

[23] Survey of London: volumes 29-30: St James Westminster, Part 1 (1960), pages 368-77.

[24] 28th September 1782, The Morning Post

[25] 3rd August 1782, The Morning Post

[26] 10th July 1781, The London Courant

[27] 18th April 1781, The Morning Post

[28] 31st January 1782, The Morning Chronicle

[29] 28th November 1783, The Morning Post

[30] The Bath Chronicle, in Lyson's Collectanea 1 (1) pages 95-96, British Library

[31] ibid

[32] Angelo 2.61 Reminiscences 1828-30, quoted in the article for James Graham in The Oxford Dictionary of National Biography, Volume 3, 2004

[33] Notes and Queries, 2nd series, ii 233, quoted in the article for James Graham in The Dictionary of National Biography, Volume 22, 1890

[34] The Bath Chronicle, in Lyson's Collectanea, op cit

[35] Robert Southey, Common Place Book, 4.360, quoted in the article for James Graham in The Oxford Dictionary of National Biography, op cit

[36] Published 9th April 1783, (British Museum 6327) quoted in Edwin A Dawes, The Great Illusionists, David and Charles, 1979, page 68

[37] The Gentleman's Magazine, Volume 52, February 1782, page 58

[38] 5th August 1788, The Aberdeen Journal

[39] 3rd-6th July 1789, The Glasgow Advertiser

[40] 24th September 1792, Aris's Birmingham Gazette

[41] 4th June 1792, Aris's Birmingham Gazette

[42] 17th December 1795, The Derby Mercury

[43] 10th December 1795, The Derby Mercury

[44] e.g. 27th August 1794, The Hereford Journal

[45] e.g. 16th July 1792 Aris's Birmingham Gazette

[46] 6th September 1793, The Shrewsbury Chronicle

[47] 27th February 1796, The Nottingham Journal; 5th November 1792, The Birmingham Gazette

[48] 27th February 1796, The Nottingham Journal; 24th September 1792, The Birmingham Gazette

[49] 2nd September 1796, The Iris or Sheffield Advertiser

[50] 13th October 1798, The Newcastle Courant

[51] 18th March 1793, Aris's Birmingham Gazette

[52] 6th September 1790, quoted in "A History of Hypnosis", Alan Gauld, Cambridge University Press, 1992, page 198

[53] 5th, 9th, 12th and 21st March 1791, The Daily Advertiser, www.british-history.ac.uk

[54] 12th November 1785, The Morning Herald

[55] 14th and 21st January 1791, The Chester Chronicle

[56] 10th December 1795, The Derby Mercury; 23rd January 1797, The York Courant

[57] 14th January 1791, The Chester Chronicle

[58] 17th March 1790, The Cumberland Pacquet

[59] 14th January 1791, The Chester Chronicle

[60] 21st December 1791, The Wolverhampton Chronicle

[61] 6th July 1790, The Manchester Mercury
[62] 16th December 1789, The Cumberland Pacquet
[63] The Dictionary of National Biography, volume 22, 1890
[64] BBC news report, 13th July 2004
[65] "Essay on Quackery", op cit
[66] e.g. 13th August 1794, The Hereford Journal

CHAPTER 3

WONDERS! WONDERS! AND WONDERS!

"Yet one cannot help wondering - but plague on it,
if I wonder any longer, my letter will be as full of wonders
as one of Katterfelto's advertisements"
Sir Walter Scott, "Redgauntlet", Letter 3, 1824

Modesty was never going to be one of Katterfelto's failings. He certainly had no inhibitions in declaring himself "the most astonishing of all Philosophers, ancient and modern".[1] In the eighteenth century, "philosophy" could mean not only rational thought about "life, the universe and everything" but also "natural philosophy" which was developing into what we know as science. Wherever he went "the Prussian Philosopher" always kept his lecture rooms "warm and properly illuminated"[2] with the help of log fires and candles. However, these were not the only source of illumination on offer. His professed aim was to enlighten the nation and whenever Katterfelto exhibited there was sure to be abundant light: physical, intellectual and even spiritual. After all, this was the age of the Enlightenment and Katterfelto was determined to be seen as a key figure within it.

The Enlightenment affected almost every part of British and western culture. At its intellectual centre was a growing confidence in the ability of human reason and observation to establish firm foundations for knowledge. Many factors had kindled it but the blue touchpaper had been lit by Sir Isaac Newton (1642-1727). Among many things in his glittering career, Newton had explained both gravity and the regular, predictable movement of the planets. These astonishing achievements showed that the mysteries of the universe really could yield to the power of human reason. The development of a scientific method for studying and explaining natural phenomena was beginning to bear fruit with exciting new discoveries in a range of fields such as optics, chemistry, magnetism and electricity, while a revolution was underway in many other spheres of thought.

In British society, as elsewhere, there was great public enthusiasm to learn about these new developments. Scotland was reasonably well placed to meet the need with its four flourishing universities, underpinned by a virtually nationwide system of parish schools and a growing number of good fee-paying ones. However, formal education in England was in a fairly parlous state. For the very rich, provided they were male, celibate and Anglican, there was Oxford or Cambridge, although even the number of these elect few had declined sharply during the century and few bothered to graduate. As for the public schools, these were viewed by Henry Fielding and others as "the nurseries of all vice and immorality". There was also a growing feeling that the Anglican grammar schools were teaching an irrelevant curriculum based on classical civilisation, rather than "modern" and "useful" subjects desired by many.

As a result, a lot of very successful people were self-taught and there was a rapidly expanding market in books by which people could improve themselves. Others could satisfy their hunger for knowledge by enrolling at one of the respected Dissenting Academies. However, many of the public relied on the academic equivalent of the medical "irregulars": namely the scientific lecturers who toured the country. Delivering wide-ranging courses of lectures, these enterprising individuals earned their living by satisfying the public's inquisitiveness and appetite for intellectual improvement.

One of the most successful of them was James Dinwiddie. Dinwiddie had begun as a maths teacher at Dumfries Academy, and later took to the high roads of Scotland, Ireland and England, lecturing on topics that included gunnery, fortification, pyrotechnics, electricity, heat, navigation, optics and astronomy. While in Dublin he also experimented with and lectured on the diving bell. In the 1790s Dinwiddie was invited by the scientifically minded George McCartney, Ambassador to China, to accompany him there as part of the British Embassy. From China he went on to teach in Bengal, before returning to London as a wealthy man.

So the popularisers of science, although usually unattached to any academic institution, were men of real knowledge and ability, and they made the rapid developments in understanding available to the general, fee paying, public. Katterfelto wanted to make it clear to his audiences that he was to be numbered among their ranks:

His Lecture every Monday evening will be on Electricity,
Tuesday on the Loadstone and Magnetism, Wednesday on the
Air Pump, Thursday on Optics, Friday on the Orrery,
Mechanical Powers and Hydraulics, Saturday on Fixed Air,
and on the Mestatic Apparatus.[3]

This was typical of the syllabus of lectures delivered by his peers. Also typical was the claim that his scientific apparatus was "very numerous and elegantly finished, and all on the newest construction, many of which are not to be equalled in Europe"[4] (and which was valued, he said, at up to £7000).[5] Despite the usual puffery, Katterfelto was not without some ability in natural philosophy. As one eyewitness recalled:

He was dressed in a black gown and square cap; his apparatus
was in excellent order, and very well managed, he conducted
every experiment with great certainty, never failing; and ...
much knowledge might be gained from his lecture.[6]

2. Woodcut of Katterfelto

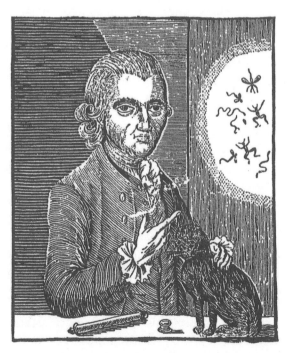

This is very much the impression given of Katterfelto in a woodcut produced in 1783, and which was described at the time as a remarkable likeness.[7] It presents him as a respectable and serious teacher: an image that must have pleased him greatly. However, in Katterfelto we have someone who was creating for himself a persona not just of any old touring lecturer but of a great philosopher, teaching things "untaught before". He also believed, perhaps rightly, that what people turned out for on a dark evening was not simply dry rational instruction but a bit of awe and wonder, and, above all, a show.

Without doubt, the centrepiece of his daytime exhibition was the solar microscope which had played such a vital part in his rise to fame as a quack. This instrument was a kind of magic lantern: a box that fitted into the shutters of a darkened room. A mirror caught the sun's rays and reflected them through a lens in the box, so as to project greatly magnified images onto a sheet or screen so that they could be viewed by many people at once.

Katterfelto constantly referred to his solar microscope as "new-invented" or "new-improved", neatly implying that it was he who had invented or improved it. However, its creator was Johannes Lieberkuhn, a German physician and anatomist, who designed it in 1739 in order to show images of specimens to large classes of anatomy students. It was then popularised in England by John Cuff, a maker of microscopes, spectacles and barometers in London, who came up with a new and improved design that was copied for many years. The solar microscope then made its way into the standard equipment of travelling lecturers. So Katterfelto's instrument was neither new in itself, nor new to the world of eighteenth century adult education. What *was* new was the way that Katterfelto used it. He was probably the first person in Britain (and certainly the most celebrated) to use the instrument to blend scientific instruction with commercial entertainment.

Katterfelto's microscope had made its first modest appearances in adverts in May and June 1781. However, it was during the flu epidemic of the following year that he began to realise its great potential. As the disease was raging he let it be known that the pernicious insects responsible "will be magnified as large as an ox, and a hundred persons may have a view at one time".[8] Given the scale of the health scare, there must have been considerable interest in seeing the culprits responsible for so many deaths, although encouraging lots of people to gather together in a warm room during a flu epidemic was, as we now know, exactly the wrong thing to be doing!

The solar microscope's revelations became a central part of Katterfelto's publicity and performances from then on.

The insects in the hedges will be seen larger than ever, and those insects which caused the late influenza will be seen as large as birds, and in a drop of water, the size of a pin head, there will be seen above 50,000 insects.[9]

These were the microorganisms that had first been discovered by Leeuwenhoek and which he had named "Animalcule". Under Katterfelto's microscope the number of creatures that could be viewed ranged from a paltry 5000 to an astounding 500,000 in a single droplet, and what a menagerie there was to see. They appeared "as rough as a bear"[10] and as large as lobsters, birds, walking sticks, eels, rats, rattlesnakes or rabbits. Some were even reminiscent of "his favourite Black Cat".[11] Two particularly interesting types were "the Wonderful WHEEL INSECTS and the SURPRIZING POLYPES."[12]

The places where these life forms were lurking multiplied as well. They could be found in "beer, vinegar, blood, flower, cheese etc. and there will be seen many surprizing insects in different vegetables and above 200 other dead objects."[13] Then there were the

50,000 live insects in a drop of Woman's Milk and also above 70,000 ... in a drop of Cow's Milk, and live insects as large as Snakes ... on the teeth, and in Matter that comes from Wounds above 60,000 in the size of a Pin's Head.[14]

If some of this was a little stomach-turning, it wasn't long before the good Doctor realised that he could give the public a demonstration "that man is a lump of corruption; for everything he eats and everything he drinks abounds with insects and thousands of maggots are shewn in a bit of cheese or meat."[15] No wonder a certain "Welch Gentleman" who had seen these insects "ran out of the room, saying he would not in future eat any more cheese were he to get £10,000 for every ounce."[16]

This particular gentleman got around a bit, turning up at Katterfelto's shows over the length and breadth of the country. For instance in Chesterfield, where "the Sublime Katterfelto was exhibiting his Arcana of Secrets", the Welshman had gone to see

a half crown's worth of Wonders but was so terrified with the
Spectacle before him that he ran off post haste in a chaise and
four to escape being devoured by the Millions of Monsters
which the Doctor, by the help of his Solar Microscope
exhibited in drops of milk, water and vinegar. Those who
doubt the authenticity of this anecdote may, if they please, be
assured of the truth from the Doctor's own lips.[17]

Our Welsh friend was not the only person to be alarmed at seeing such greatly magnified images of what their food and drink contained. Many of "the first Ladies and Gentlemen" in Liverpool, Mansfield and elsewhere were also reported to have been shocked. Some degree of concern, or at least morbid fascination, at these microscopic life forms may well have been genuine. The same could be said about the reaction to the Doctor's revelations concerning the creatures that he found living in the wig-powder worn by the fashionable:

It is proved, he says, that those ladies and gentlemen who
wear old Mareschal powder in their hair, have a larger army
in their heads than the King has now by land and sea. From
such wonders, such armies, and such heads who could not wish
to be delivered.[18]

Fortunately deliverance *was* at hand, once again through the solar microscope. The wonderful instrument revealed "how the Spirits kill the insects", or in other words the disinfecting power of alcohol. This remedy to the insect plague meant that Katterfelto was also able to help gentlemen gardeners "to preserve Flowers, Trees and Vegetables from Insects and Destruction in Gardens and Hot-houses".[19] (His gardening tips also included "how to forward various flowers and lilies, and to preserve the blossom of trees.")[20] Farmers, butchers and sheep dealers would also be greatly advantaged by this new miracle cure, providing that they spent five shillings on a bottle of tincture to kill "the Insects that are on a Sheep's Liver that causes the Rot".[21]

Despite occasional moments of revulsion at the ubiquitous nature of these previously invisible life forms, his solar microscope opened "a new world in miniature", and the proper reaction to this should be one of awe and wonder. The people of London were soon being invited to witness "The most wonderful, surprising and astonishing great Wonders and Wonders of Nature, which are beyond all description".[22] Indeed it was not long before this microscopic world had provided Katterfelto with his most famous catchphrase: "WONDERS! WONDERS! and WONDERS!" which introduced many of his adverts for the rest of his life. Sometimes he got so carried away by these insights into the natural world that he proclaimed four, five or even six-fold "Wonders!"

His relentless promotional material drove his catchphrase home. All of a sudden it seemed that everything was wonderful. The microscope that made these revelations possible was itself "surprising and wonderful" (the like of which "may never be seen again for a century to come").[23] Likewise, it was natural to conclude that the man who was bringing all these wonders before the public must be none other than "the Wonder of Wonders".[24] Not surprisingly the plaudits poured in:

> Great Nature's wonders are by thee displayed
> In various forms, as they are various made.
> In different liquids where the nicest eye
> Cannot the least of active life espy,
> You by your Microscope, bring forth to view,
> With every part enlarged, yet justly true.
> Herbs, Insects and Animalculas appear
> Beyond what all description can declare
> Sense stands astonished at the wond'rous sight,
> And every thinking man must feel delight![25]

Katterfelto was by no means the first to claim to offer great wonders to the world. For example, "the Wonder of Wonders" was already a well-worn phrase. During the seventeenth century numerous pamphlets were published announcing some incredible event as the Wonder of Wonders: there was "strange news from Newton in Yorkshire - being a relation of a gentleman turned into a statue of stone" and "two old men how [sic] come invisibly to Rome and their ten strange prophecies"; and who could forget the 1726 classic of a woman near Guildford who was "delivered lately of seventeen Rabbets, and three legs of a Tabby Cat etc".[26]

During the 1720s, Jonathan Swift (author of Gulliver's Travels) took up the theme in a series of tracts satirising this sort of hot air. For Swift "the Wonderful Wonder of Wonders" was so much flatulence, consisting of such things as "an accurate description of the birth, education, manner of living, religion, politicks, learning etc. of mine a-se".[27] He also issued a satirical advert for a fictitious conjurer by the name of "Schoritz". This proclaimed "The Wonder of all the Wonders that ever the World Wondered at"; wonders that included such things as giving "any Gentlemen leave to drive forty twelvepenny nails up to the head in a porter's backside, and then place the said porter in a loadstone [i.e. magnetic] chair, which draws out every nail, and the porter feels no pain".[28]

As in other things, therefore, Katterfelto was not all that original in his catchphrase and perhaps unwittingly he had chosen one that had strong satirical associations. One person who joined the growing queue to lampoon Katterfelto for his scientific (as well as his medical) hot air was William Blake. Blake's work was not all art and "Jerusalem". Among many pieces of writing is a satire from the mid-1780s featuring three philosophers who engage in nonsensical discussions. They are joined by "Inflammable Gass the Windfinder", who has "a bottle of air that could spread a Plague". Being invited to show the assembly his microscopic experiments he begins to hold forth:

> *"Here ladies and gentlemen" he said, "I'll shew you a louse, or a flea, or a butterfly, or a cockchafer, the blade bone of a tittleback. No, No. Here's a bottle of wind that I took up in the boghouse."*

Calamity followed when Inflammable Gass broke the bottle of wind and let out the Pestilence. Running from the room he cried out:

> *"Come out! Come out! We are putrefied! We are corrupted! Our lungs are destroy'd with the Flogiston. This will spread a plague thro' the Island!" He was downstairs the very first. On the back of him came all the others in a heap.*[29]

Other satirists picked up Katterfelto's catch phrase and included "wonders" in one form or another in the various cartoons of him. Commercial outlets also began to take notice and rode the wave of his notoriety. The greatest flattery is imitation (even if flavoured with a hint of mockery) so we can imagine Katterfelto having a satisfied smile on his face when he opened his newspaper on Christmas Day 1782 to read that "WONDERS of WONDERS! and the GREATEST of all WONDERS!" were now to be seen not only at Spring Gardens but also at Bryant's Cloak Warehouse, which was selling "strong, serviceable, warm and comfortable great coats for winter wear".[30]

All this awe and wonder was not merely a route to fame but also to true piety as well. Newton and his fellow scientists were clear that the laws of nature which they were discovering were nothing less than expressions of God's providential will for the universe. As a "divine and moral philosopher" Katterfelto took the same view: he was setting before the public nothing less than "the wonderful works of Providence".

Strange Wonders hid from human sight,
His Microscope can bring to light,
The works of God, unseen by eyes,
The means of seeing, this supplies,
All haste to him, whilst here he stayes,
Then sing, like me, the Doctor's Praise.
    W. Witty *A LOVER OF PHILOSOPHY*[31]

For Katterfelto, it was his religious duty to call people to come and see "the most wonderful Exhibition in the World", and his call was rich with gospel overtones: "He who has eyes to see, let him see!"[32]In seeing these wonders they were honouring their Maker and receiving enlightenment, while those who failed to come did "offend their Maker"[33] and condemned themselves to live in the darkness of ignorance:

All persons on earth, even the most religious, live in darkness
in this world if they are able to see but won't see those great
wonderful works of our Maker.[34]

And when he said that all persons lived in darkness, he meant all persons, including:

The Signor, His Holiness the Pope, The Great Emperor,
Kings, Queens and Princes in Europe, likewise all the
Bishops, Clergy and different Preachers; the Masonic
gentlemen, Professors of the Faculty, and all other Sons of
Knowledge, and such that go by the name of being
religious...if they are able but will not spare and find time to
see the most surprising and astonishing Solar Microscope
Exhibition.[35]

55

The unparalleled enlightenment on offer was clear "particularly in the polite circles", where it had become common to ask:

'Have you seen the Solar Microscope Exhibition?' If an answer 'No' is returned, the reply is 'Then you have seen Nothing'.[36]

To ram the point home, his lecture on optics, which explained "the eye's formation, mechanism divine",[37] was adapted to rail against "all such Persons that are not totally blind, but will not see."[38]

It was not long before Katterfelto's new marketing ploy brought forth another line in satire. In July 1782 the Haymarket Theatre began staging a pantomime by the name of "None are so Blind as those who won't see", of which the central character was one "Dr. Catterpillar". The farce was written by Charles Dibbin with music by Samuel Arnold, a pairing who staged many late eighteenth century productions. They had already produced one that lampooned Dr. James Graham called "The Genius of Nonsense", which was advertised as "an Original, Whimsical, Operatical, Pantomimical, Farcical, Electrical, Naval, Military, Temporary, Local Extravaganza".[39] It had featured "the Emperor of the Quacks" and "the Goddess of Health", along with "Views of the Temple of Health"; books of the songs could even be bought on the way out of the theatre. Graham had been incensed and had tried, without success, to buy a copy of the stage bill in order to mount a libel action.

Katterfelto also took up arms against Dibbin's scurrilous attack on his reputation, but he did so in print rather than in the courts:

If Dr Catterpillar, or Mr Red Stocking, or Mr Big Wig, or Mr Little Wit, could exhibit the Solar Microscope on the stage ... without Sun in the evening, he would surprise the learned and instruct the ignorant; and then Dr Caterpillar would exceed Mr Katterfelto, and all other ingenious Philosophers in the world.[40]

He even took off the very characters that were poking fun at him, with the help of some projected images of the stars of the show, to which he added his own impersonations:

All those Dramatic Persons who did appear on the stage at the

Theatre in the Hay-market, will be seen at Mr Katterfelto's
Exhibition Room, by Optics, every one in their character; and
Mr Katterfelto intends to take off every one in the farce of
"None are so Blind as those who won't see" particularly Dr
Catterpillar, likewise Commodore Barnacle, Valentine
Porpoise ... with great improvements of other Characters.[41]

Fortunately Katterfelto was not left alone to fight in defence of his good name. Another supposed member of his fan club, "Dr Hamily", a fairly regular contributor to his advertisements, came to his aid attacking the way "venal puppets of the mimic stage" ridiculed the great philosopher:

When dearth of wit begets dull pantomime,
Applause to reach, they on thy merits climb,
Seek crowded houses from thy well-known name,
And on thy talents raise a borrow'd fame ...
And thus the mimic when he hears applause,
Forgets thy merit is the real cause.[42]

After his failed attempt to sue for libel, Dr. Graham chose to ignore the continued mockery of him on the stage. Katterfelto on the other hand kept returning to his own detractors in his advertisements. Indeed, more than five years after he had left London he was still referring to the satire "None are so blind".[43] This might give the impression that it had touched a nerve: that either his ego or his reputation had been quite hurt by it. However, it was probably just that the farce, and his repeated drawing attention to it in the papers, helped to keep him in the public eye. Once again, he knew that there was no such thing as bad publicity.

He certainly needed all the help he could get. Sometimes it was simply apathy on the public's part, perhaps fuelled by the satires, which prevented them seeing the wonders on display. However, the British weather also played its part. To give clear definition of fine details, and to show what Katterfelto called "the Animality in the Air", the solar microscope required very strong sunlight: a "fair Sunshiney Day" as he put it.[44] As and when the sun didn't shine, or when it was too dim, Katterfelto could always fall back on his "new-improved Compound Microscope" instead. However, this more familiar form of microscope had one big draw back for the showman, in that it limited viewing of the slides to one person at a time.

Therefore, physical light was crucial to Katterfelto's enterprise of bringing mental and spiritual enlightenment to the world. In London, he explained that it was a lack of light (but was it really a lack of money?) that led him to move from Cox's Museum: firstly to 228, High Holborn and then to 22 (and finally 24), Piccadilly. Similarly, on his travels, when choosing a room in a hostelry for his exhibition he would, wherever possible, opt for one with a good south-facing aspect.

As it turned out, Katterfelto could not have picked a worse time to launch his weather-dependent wonders on the world. The summer of 1783 was exceptionally stormy: "No year in man's memory ever abounded more with tempestuous weather, hurricanes, etc than the present".[45] And much worse was to come. Between June 1783 and February 1784, the largest series of volcanic eruptions in the northern hemisphere for a thousand years took place in Iceland. Mount Laki's eruptions created the world's largest lava flow covering five hundred square kilometres, and pumped over a hundred million tons of toxic gas into the atmosphere. Not only did nine thousand Icelanders perish along with livestock and vegetation, but also the gases in the atmosphere reflected sunlight back out to space, drastically reducing the amount of light for several years. Downwind, in Britain and northern Europe, low-level gases brought "dry fogs" for months afterwards and there were three years of exceptionally cold winters; the coldest in five hundred years in some places. (The effects were even felt as far away as Egypt, which suffered a severe famine.)

So, through these years and beyond, Katterfelto had to get used to prolonged periods of bad weather. These were seriously bad news for him and often brought forth the following lament:

The Sun has been very inauspicious to that phenomenon of genius and star of philosophy Dr Katterfelto since his arrival among us; twice only has this great man had the felicity of uncorking his vinegar bottle [to clean the microscope's lense] in the course of a fortnight; niggardly Sol, as if envious of the Doctor's rays, having withdrawn his influence. Hence the philosopher's face, like the sun, is rather clouded and the splendid beams of his imagination are obscured by the vapors of the atmosphere; ... if Phoebus [i.e. Apollo, the Greek god of the Sun] kindly undraws her veil the Doctor will again open the door of his new world of wonders![46]

Although the cloudy weather might spoil the show, it could not dampen his humour or his hope. In Chester it had

a very serious effect on the sublime Doctor Katterfelto and his colleagues since their arrival among us. His black cat has lost much of her wonted powers – his flea has had a severe touch of the rheumatics – his louse has been troubled with a slight influenza attended with a cough – several of his insects are dead of a bilious cholic – and the Doctor himself to complete the catalogue of maladies is a little feverish – The rays of the Sun, however, may yet effect a wonderful renovation.[47]

Eventually the ever-inventive philosopher found a solution to this regular lack of the sun in the British Isles, announcing to the residents of Derby "his Lunary Microscope (but called Solar in the day time)" which was powered by "a new-invented strong light" that burnt "without the help of oil, tallow or spirits".[48]

This strong light was none other than white phosphorus. It had been discovered in 1669 by a German merchant, Henning Brand, who had been boiling putrefied urine. The reason for this rather unpleasant sounding activity was that, like most chemists of his day, Brand was pursuing the alchemist's dream of creating gold. Although disappointed in his search, he succeeded in isolating the first element to be discovered since ancient times. While some chemists began to study the properties of phosphorus in more detail (discovering that it could also be extracted from bone), and medical practitioners began to administer it, along with its toxic side-effects, to their patients, others began to exploit its remarkable properties of glowing in contact with air and of igniting at about forty degrees centigrade. This suggested the name "phosphorus", from the Greek for "light-bringer". Given the close similarity in meaning to "Lucifer", or "light-bearer", as well as the mysterious and almost unimaginable ability phosphorus had to create fire on demand, it later became known as "the Devil's Element". A new source of fire also suggested a variety of commercial opportunities, which merely awaited an inventor with the necessary entrepreneurial talent.

Within little more than a decade, Robert Boyle had covered a piece of paper with this new wonder element, had rubbed it with a small piece of wood coated with sulphur, and fire resulted. Although friction matches as we know them would have to wait until 1827 for John Walker, an English Chemist and Apothecary, to coat a stick with the necessary chemicals, "Phosphorick Matches" were being advertised for sale in London as early as 1782. For example, those made in Paris by Messrs Bettally and Nose were being sold by Mr. Ramsden, an Optician from Piccadilly, together with instructions to: "break off the point and expose to the air and they immediately light themselves".[49]

True to form, Londoners were soon being informed that in fact "Dr Katterfelto is the real inventor of the Phosphorous Matches".[50] However, within weeks Katterfelto was advertising a far superior product: what he called his "new-invented alarum".

> *It is far better than the phosphoric matches, which have been boasted of so much in the newspapers for these twelve months past, those phosphoric matches having been found to miss very often, but Dr Katterfelto's invention never does.*[51]

Compared to these matches (which in fact he kept on making and selling)[52] his alarum was ten times cheaper, far more effective, and did not "lose [its] virtue for twenty years, by sea or land".[53] It was also good for firing off cannons, pistols or blunderbusses without the usual need for "flint, steel or fire".[54] It would even protect the nation's health, because this new "Light and Fire"

> *is also a very great benefit in a Room or Town where there is a dangerous Fever, Plague or Pestilence, also in a House or Gaol, where there is a Quantity of foul Air, as it will purify the Air.*[55]

In other words, his phosphorus-based alarum would drive out the miasmas along with the many forms of disease they were believed to carry. This meant that it would be of great value in bedchambers when people were suffering from "asthmatic complaints and violent pains on their breath etc";[56] Katterfelto was pleased to report that it had already saved over forty lives in the city of Dublin.[57]

Phosphorus was a chemical wonder and he made the most of it throughout his travels. It featured heavily in Katterfelto's chemistry lectures.[58] He demonstrated how to make up to "seven different kinds" of the element;[59] sold it in solid, liquid, powder and "aether" forms, to a public that was fascinated by the new substance;[60] and it may have been the secret ingredient in other "newly invented" merchandise, such as his "Fire Machines".[61] So it was, that in later years it came to his rescue as a "new-invented strong light" when the sun refused to shine for his solar microscope.

The risk of a lack of sunlight affecting his exhibitions led to an alternative and very topical solution being suggested during his visit to York in 1797:

> *Several of the London papers, these fourteen days past, have expressed that the noted Prussian Philosopher, Dr Katterfelto, in this City was making a pair of Bellows to blow the clouds away if they came before his Grand Solar Microscope! If so, we have great reason to believe that the above great philosopher, being a well-wisher to Great Britain, will likewise blow the French fleet from Hull, if they offer to make a landing there, or on any part of the coast.*[62]

Here Katterfelto's wit was connecting with current events. At the time there was considerable concern about a possible invasion following the French Revolution. The threat had begun in 1793 when, following the execution of Louis XVI, France had declared war on Britain. The papers were currently reporting that the French fleet had suffered greatly from bad weather on an Irish expedition. The ships had made it back to port in a fairly shattered state and were being repaired in haste for some new military venture.

Ever the opportunist, war provided Katterfelto with another means to attract the paying public. In 1795, he let it be known that his audiences could see "by the help of Optics as Natural as life, AN ENGLISH FLEET in a hot Engagement with the FRENCH".[63]Undoubtedly, Katterfelto was presenting this as an image of the sea battle known as the "Glorious First of June". This was the first major sea battle of the war and had taken place on that date in 1794. In it, Admiral Earl Howe, who commanded his force from an armchair on the quarterdeck of his ship, had succeeded in routing the French while sinking one and capturing six of their ships. The victory was widely celebrated in Britain and, like so many others before and since, was enshrined in many works of art. Some of these were as small as four inches across. It was probably one of these that Katterfelto was projecting onto the big screen.

Likewise, back in 1792 the residents of Birmingham had been invited to view a scene from a battle against a joint French and Spanish fleet.[64] There hadn't been such a battle since 1744 during the colourfully named "War of Jenkins's Ear" (begun after Captain

Robert Jenkins had appeared in Parliament brandishing his ear, which he claimed had been severed by the Spanish). Nevertheless, Katterfelto was probably bothered less with historical accuracy than with capitalising on the old enmity with France and Spain and exploiting the patriotic feelings of the time.

As well as scenes of war, Katterfelto showed people a vast range of transparent paintings on glass and silk: "50,000 different optical Figures and different Characters from the Grand Signor to the Beggar, nearly as large as life".[65] All these various images were projected via what he called his "Royal Patent Delineator". This was a kind of camera obscura which William Storer, an English instrument maker, had produced in 1778. It was far superior to its predecessors, creating a more brilliant picture and much clearer focus. Storer called it the "Royal Accurate Delineator". Katterfelto was happy to change the name and claim it as his own.

Nor was Katterfelto alone in combining paintings and optical equipment to bring new visual experiences to the public. Magic lanterns had been around since at least the 1670s, but at first their use had been restricted to the home or laboratory. However, with better lenses and light sources came the possibility of using instruments like these in front of larger audiences. With all his different optical wonders, Katterfelto played a significant part in this movement, which was bringing mass entertainment to the big screen for the first time.

Two of the great optical shows in London at the time were Sir Ashton Lever's "Holophusicon" and Philip James de Loutherbourg's "Eidophusikon". The latter used mirrors and pulleys to show "Moving Pictures" of such "phenomena of nature" as the Cataract of Niagara, "the rising of the moon with a water spout off the coast of Japan", and "Satan straying his troops on the banks of the fiery lake".[66] Loutherbourg also used his artistic skills in the service of David Garrick's theatre, creating innovative set designs that astounded the public with a moon that rose in the sky and leaves that changed colours. (He was also a skilled painter of miniatures and could well have been the originator of Katterfelto's naval pictures.)

Another screen phenomenon in London and the provinces was "the Ombres Chinoise" or "Les Ombres Anglois".[67] This was a version of traditional Chinese shadow puppets, which had been introduced to Paris in 1776 by the French puppeteer Dominique Séraphin. It quickly spread to Britain and became an overnight success, entertaining audiences for many years with a wide range of moralistic and comic tales, such as "The Spanish House-breakers, who by their crafty Contrivance, lived on their plunder for several years".[68]

The various screen attractions, of Katterfelto and others, blended entertainment and education, light and enlightenment, and seem to symbolise an age full of wonders and wondering. With "diversification" as his watchword, Katterfelto offered more than his fair share of curiosities to his wondering public. While on sunny days they might witness his Solar Microscope Exhibition hourly from 10am to 4pm, on cloudy days their disappointment could be offset by viewing his Grand Museum hourly from 9am to 7pm.[69]

This museum consisted of "Paintings, various Mechanical Powers and Natural History" and included "as many, or more, curious articles (which he has collected in his 26 years Travels) than have been seen in Sir Ashton Lever's, Cox's, or the British Museum in London, or the Grand Museum in Paris."[70] Among the hundreds of natural phenomena that Katterfelto had on display were fossils and agates collected from the Yorkshire coast[71] and "a few of the finest diamond beetles".[72] Diamond Beetles, or "Botany Bay Weevils" as they are also known, were among the first insects described by the great naturalist Joseph Banks when he landed at the said bay along with Captain Cook in 1770. In this culture of curiosity, the previously unknown flora and fauna of the antipodes, Diamond Beetles among them, soon became another of the fascinations of the moment. Once again, Katterfelto cashed in by offering them for sale.

So much for the daytime. In the evenings he presented his course of between six and sixteen lectures. These were on a whole range of "interesting, important, instructive and entertaining subjects, viz – on the general properties of Matter, Mechanics, Pneumatics, Chymistry, Electricity, Hydrostatics, Optics, Gravitation, Magnetism and Astronomy".[73] Astronomy was, naturally enough, a favourite for Katterfelto's evening performances and was accompanied by further sophisticated equipment. The indispensable tool of the astronomer's trade was of course the telescope, and those who came to view it occasionally received

> a ticket (given gratis) to see the spots in the Sun and the mountains in the Moon, and some other Heavenly Bodies by his large Reflecting Telescope, which is as good a one as in the three Kingdoms.[74]

With the help of this magnificent instrument he was able to show "the GOODNESS of the Sun, Moon and other Planets", [75] and to open the minds of people who

> *may think the Stars are out of his reach, yet if they will attend his evening lecture … they will soon find that Jupiter, Mars and Saturn and the rest of the Gents above, not forgetting the Great Bear, are old acquaintances of the Doctor's![76]*

One spectacular opportunity to use his telescope arose during his stay in Liverpool during 1791. In the early afternoon of the 3rd April "several learned and principal Gentlemen" gathered at the Golden Lion Inn on Dale Street. They had come to witness one of nature's heavenly wonders, and they were in for a treat. They entered a darkened exhibition room in which three pieces of scientific equipment were arranged: "Doctor Katterfelto's Patent Delineator, also…his large Reflecting Telescope and new-invented Solar Microscope." On the wall opposite was a large sheet onto which the instruments were projecting three distinct images of the sun. Just before one o'clock the images began to change dramatically. An annular eclipse of the sun was taking place. The moon was passing in front of the sun but it was too far away from the earth to block out the sun completely. Instead, the outer layers of the sun were still visible as a brilliant ring, or annulus, surrounding the moon. Those attending Katterfelto's exhibition that afternoon were able to view the spectacle safely, "to the greatest advantage" and in triplicate. Over the next couple of weeks Katterfelto was also able to announce that during this particular eclipse he had been able to make some new "discoveries" that would add further lustre to his already astronomical reputation.[77]

Then, as now, astronomers sought not only to show people the heavens but also to explain them. Since the early eighteenth century this had been aided by another vital piece of equipment: an orrery. Increasing skills in engineering and craftsmanship meant that Newton's mechanical view of the universe could now be illustrated by this device. It was named after Charles Boye, 4th Earl of Cork and Orrery in Ireland, who had been given one of the first such machines by a clockmaker. By use of a clockwork mechanism the orrery showed how the Earth, Moon and planets (as far out as Saturn) moved in orbits around the Sun. It was an expensive item and highly sought after by the aristocracy. It was also *de rigueur* for a touring scientific lecturer.

Katterfelto was no exception. With this visual aid he explained the reasons for eclipses such as that witnessed at Liverpool, but also the cause of the changing seasons, the cycle of day and night, the movement of the planets, the gravitational effect of the heavenly bodies on the earth and so on. All these were part of Katterfelto's lecture programme, and they gave substance to his hope that instead of frittering away their time and money on frivolous forms of entertainment, "every Person this Year would learn the Distance and Size of the Sun, Moon and Earth and … the Size and Distance of Mercury and the Planets next year."[78]

Whether it was daytime or night, whether people were coming to see his Solar Microscope Exhibition or to peer at the heavens, to view his Grand Museum or to attend his course of Lectures, Mr. Katterfelto desired that every man of every profession should be interested "in the riches which the Doctor brings from darkness to light."[79] In particular, there was one body of men whom Katterfelto hoped would have a special interest in his "Dark Secret Wonders": the Freemasons.

After leaving London, Katterfelto arrived in Norwich where he added another dimension to his persona. He became, for the first time, "Brother Katterfelto". Here he lectured "by particular desire of the most ancient and honourable Free and accepted Masons of the City". He appealed to his fellow Masons to come from forty miles around to see his "occult" secrets; (in this period "occult" simply meant "hidden"). These were secrets which had already enlightened "the Grand Lodges at London, Dublin, Edinburgh, Berlin, Copenhagen, Stockholm, Petersburgh, Paris, Vienna, Dresden and several other Lodges in Europe".[80] With an eye to masonry (of one kind or another) he included a lecture on architecture,[81] and also exhibited "various sympathetical clocks, which have surprised all the Masters of the ancient and modern lodges" of Europe;[82] (what he elsewhere called "Masonical Clocks").[83]

By now there were lodges in all the major towns and cities of Britain, and to many of these Brother Katterfelto made his appeal. He often did so with the help of "the rule of 9", trusting that the Gentlemen Craftsmen would follow its instruction and favour him with their company.[84] In Manchester, he offered to enlighten the "Sons of Knowledge" with lectures that "all such Members that are Sons of the East will find it worthy of their notice".[85] Likewise, the Masons of Nottingham found that he would

spare no pains to oblige or instruct, to entertain or surprise, the Curious; as on this night he promises to reveal something which will be confessedly ... of the utmost consequence to the above Honourable and Useful MASONIC SOCIETIES.[86]

In Birmingham, the Doctor promised to display some experiments

which have given the highest Satisfaction to His Majesty the Prince of Wales now the grand Master of the Masons in England. Brother Katterfelto will receive at the Door, Brethren by the Rule of Masonry, in a friendly brotherly Manner.[87]

Once again though, appearances were deceptive. In truth, the hidden knowledge that the Doctor was imparting was not something restricted to the Craft. Rather it concerned the same wonders of the natural world that he had been revealing in his lectures and exhibition over the years. Frequently, as at Norwich, Katterfelto only appealed to the Brethren towards the end of his stay. This suggests that his supposed Masonic connections were only being brought into the light as a way of trying to redress flagging audience figures. That Katterfelto was using Masonry, rather than being a true initiate into its mysteries, became clear in Sheffield where he invited Freemasons to come and see him "disentangle your system of blunders".[88]This must have taken some nerve, given that he was actually using the Masonic lodge in the town for his performances (as he also did in Newcastle).

In a modern context it may seem strange that Katterfelto was able to perform in the lodges and open them to the general public. However, Masonry in this period had not retreated behind as thick a veil of secrecy as in later years. It began to permeate popular culture from the 1720s onwards and was well suited to the needs of a society coming to terms with the effects of the Enlightenment. The Age of Reason had destroyed much of the power of the ancient myths. Masonry was attempting to build a new mythology, based not on superstition, but upon the moral and physical laws of the Newtonian universe. For Freemasons, although their particular brand of knowledge remained shrouded in mysteries that could only be accessed by the initiated, they were committed to proclaiming that they possessed such a secret.[89]

One example of this relative openness was William Preston's four-volume work entitled "Illustrations of Masonry". In this, any interested reader could discover:

1. A Vindication of Masonry and a demonstration of its Excellency. 2. An Illustration of the Lectures in the different Degrees, and of the Ceremonies observed at the Constitution and Consecration of Lodges, Installation of Offices …3. The Principals of Masonry explained. 4. The History of Masonry.[90]

Whatever Katterfelto's precise relationship to the Craft, there was one final aspect of his shows which he explicitly linked to Masonry and its temples: fireworks. In both Birmingham and Edinburgh audiences were treated to

a new-invented, grand and curious set of ITALIAN FIRE WORKS which have been exhibited before many of the Sovereigns of Europe, without Smoke or Smell – Various Copies of the grand Temples and Buildings of all Sorts will be seen by these Fire Works; also Solomon's Temple and a great Piece of Masonry, all in six different Colours.[91]

That Katterfelto's fireworks were heralded as Italian is no surprise. Although by the eighteenth century Germany had launched itself very successfully into the world of pyrotechnics, it was Italy that had really turned fireworks into an art form, developing shells that flew skyward and exploded in fountains of colour. Fireworks had fascinated the British since Elizabethan times, when the Queen even went so far as to create the position of "Fire Master of England". Katterfelto had a good sense of what his audiences liked and was adding value to his shows with a spectacular finale.

Wonders indeed, and how apt they were: fireworks to accompany microscopes, telescope and the illuminating power of phosphorus; lights in the darkness, from one whose mission in life was to bring intellectual, moral and spiritual enlightenment. However, as his audiences soon discovered, for all this light and enlightenment, there was also "something of the night" about this man; something dark, mysterious and not altogether natural.

---

[1] 28th July 1783, The Morning Post
[2] 3rd February 1781, The Morning Chronicle
[3] 28th March 1781, The Morning Chronicle
[4] 6th March 1782, The Morning Post

[5] 14th-17th August 1787, The Edinburgh Advertiser

[6] The Mirror of Literature, Amusement, and Instruction, op cit

[7] The European Magazine, op cit

[8] 18th April 1782, The Morning Herald

[9] 15th July 1782, The Morning Post

[10] 29th May 1782, The Morning Chronicle

[11] 18th February 1791, The York Courant

[12] 19th March 1796, The Nottingham Journal

[13] 15th July 1782, The Morning Post

[14] 2nd July 1792, Aris's Birmingham Gazette

[15] 6th June 1783, The General Advertiser, op cit

[16] 20th March 1797, The York Courant

[17] 19th August 1796, The Iris or Sheffield Advertiser

[18] 21st May 1795, Berrow's Worcester Journal

[19] 20th February 1792, Aris's Birmingham Gazette

[20] 9th April 1796, The Nottingham Journal

[21] 4th March 1793, Aris's Birmingham Gazette

[22] 17th August 1782, The Morning Post

[23] 18th April 1791, Williamson's Liverpool Advertiser

[24] 8th August 1782, The Morning Post

[25] 14th April 1790, The Cumberland Pacquet

[26] See "Wonder of wonders" in the British Library catalogue.

[27] ibid

[28] Edwin A Dawes, op cit, page 48

[29] "An Island in the Moon" in William Blake, Complete Writings, ed. Geoffrey Keynes, OUP, 1972, page 46

[30] 25th December 1782, The Morning Post

[31] 17th March 1790, The Cumberland Pacquet

[32] 28th July 1783, The Morning Post

[33] 17th February 1790, The Cumberland Pacquet

[34] 29th September 1783, The Morning Chronicle

[35] 26th November 1795, The Derby Mercury

[36] 23rd April 1795, Berrow's Worcester Journal

[37] 5th April 1781, The Morning Post

[38] 16th July 1792, Aris's Birmingham Gazette

[39] 2nd September 1780, The Morning Post

[40] 30th July 1782, The Morning Post

[41] 29th August 1782, The Morning Post

[42] 31st August 1782, The Morning Post

[43] 23rd January 1787, The York Courant; 24th February 1790, The Cumberland Pacquet

[44] 14th May 1792, Aris's Birmingham Gazette

[45] The Gentleman's Magazine, Volume 53, September 1783, page 727

[46] e.g. 29th October 1795, The Derby Mercury

[47] 14th January 1791, The Chester Chronicle
[48] 3rd December 1795, The Derby Mercury
[49] 18th April 1783, The Morning Post
[50] 8th July 1783, The General Advertiser, op cit
[51] 30th August 1783, The General Advertiser, op cit
[52] 28th August 1783, The Morning Post
[53] 28th August 1783, The Morning Post and 30th August 1783, The General Advertiser, op cit
[54] 9th October 1783, The General Advertiser, op cit
[55] 19th November 1792, Aris's Birmingham Gazette; 27th February 1796, The Nottingham Journal
[56] 3rd December 1795, The Derby Mercury
[57] 13th February 1784, The General Advertiser, op cit
[58] 5th January 1788, The Caledonian Mercury
[59] e.g. 10th August 1790, The Manchester Mercury
[60] e.g. 14th March 1791, Williamson's Liverpool Advertiser
[61] 10th December 1792, Aris's Birmingham Gazette
[62] 20th February 1797, The York Courant
[63] 28th May 1795, Berrow's Worcester Journal
[64] 16th July 1792, Aris's Birmingham Gazette
[65] 16th July 1792, also 17th and 24th September 1792, Aris's Birmingham Gazette
[66] 5th May 1783, The Morning Herald
[67] 23rd April 1783, The Daily Advertiser
[68] 9th September 1777, The Leeds Intelligencer
[69] 3rd-6th July 1789 The Glasgow Advertiser
[70] 27th January 1790, The Cumberland Pacquet
[71] Article on Katterfelto in The Dictionary of National Biography, Volume 22, 1890
[72] 30th August 1783, The General Advertiser, op cit
[73] 28th February 1791, Williamson's Liverpool Advertiser
[74] 28th July-4th August, 1789, The Glasgow Mercury
[75] 20th February 1796, The Nottingham Journal
[76] 29th October 1795, The Derby Mercury
[77] 4th and 25th April 1791, Williamson's Liverpool Advertiser
[78] 25th February 1793, Aris's Birmingham Gazette
[79] 26th August 1796, The Iris or Sheffield Advertiser
[80] 8th January 1785, The Norfolk Chronicle
[81] 8th January 1785 The Norfolk Chronicle
[82] 8th January 1785 The Norfolk Chronicle
[83] 19th November 1795, The Derby Mercury
[84] e.g. 19th November 1795, The Derby Mercury
[85] 3rd August 1790, The Manchester Mercury
[86] 13th February 1796, The Nottingham Journal
[87] 21st May 1792, Aris's Birmingham Gazette
[88] 27th September 1796, The Sheffield Courant

[89] J. Money, Experience and Identity, Manchester University Press, 1977, page 140

[90] 20th-22nd January 1784, The London Chronicle

[91] 16th July 1792, also 17th and 24th September 1792, Aris's Birmingham Gazette; 12th January 1788, The Caledonian Mercury

CHAPTER 4

THE DEVIL AND HIS IMPS

Sorcerer:
magician, thaumaturgist, theurgist, conjuror, necromancer, seer...
warlock, charmer, exorcist, mage, cunningman, medicine man...
Katerfelto, Cagliostro, Mesmer, Rosicrucian ...
Roget's Thesaurus, 1911 edition

For all his infamy as a quack and all his wonderful revelations of the microscopic world, the aspect of Katterfelto's shows that actually gained him lasting respect was magic. More than anyone else it has been the conjuring fraternity which has kept the name of Katterfelto from disappearing into the mists of time. In the early twentieth century no lesser exponent of the art than Harry Houdini described Katterfelto as "one of the most interesting characters in the history of magic".[1] True, he did also call him "a loveable vagabond" who was "bombastic in the extreme". However, Katterfelto's skills as a magician were real and considerable and were recognised as such by many in his day and since.

They were also recognised by himself of course and, true to form, Katterfelto was not embarrassed about claiming to be "the cleverest conjuror in the whole world".[2] Unlike most of his other puffs, this one had at least an outside chance of being true. He certainly showed what he called "some of the most capital feats in dexterity of hand",[3] using a whole range of the standard magical props of his day such as dice, cards, billiards, letters, money, watches, medals, clocks, silver and gold boxes, "pyramidical glasses", pistols, lemons, rings and even tennis (a highly fashionable game at the time).[4]

One reliable witness to Katterfelto's skills was that young boy in Durham who had been taken behind the stage curtain to meet the family, on the night when the deluge of rain had spoilt the performance. Fortunately, the following evening was dry:

71

On the next night of the Doctor's appearance he had a tolerably respectable auditory, and the following incidents...occasioned much laughter at the moment. Among the company was the Rev. Mr. P., a minor canon. The conjuror, in the course of his tricks, desired a card to be drawn from the pack, by one of the company, which was done, the card examined and returned into the pack, in the presence of the audience; but on the company being requested to take the card again from the pack, it could not be found. The Doctor said it must have been taken out by some one present, and civilly begged the reverend gentleman to search his pockets. Indignant at such an insinuation, the inflamed divine for some time refused to comply, but at length being persuaded, he drew forth the identical card, much to his own surprise and the amusement of the spectators. A similar trick was also played with some money, which unaccountably found its way into the reverend gentleman's pocket, a circumstance which put him out of all patience; and he proceeded most sternly to lecture the astounded Doctor for having practised his levity on a gentleman of his cloth, upon which, and threatening the poor conjuror with vengeance, he strode out of the room. Katerfelto declared that, although he was a conjuror, he did not know the gentleman was a divine.[5]

With a career spanning the last third of the eighteenth century Katterfelto was performing at a significant time in the history of magic, when various trends were coming together to help transform the public's perception of conjuring and conjurors.

Back in the late sixteenth century conjurors had been viewed as "ruffians, blasphemers, thieves, vagabonds, Jews, Turks, heretics, pagans and sorcerers."[6] It would be a long journey before magic could leave behind the twin taints of the dark arts and criminality. The first steps were taken in 1584. At a time when witches could still be executed, a man called Reginald Scot wrote a book called "The Discoverie of Witchcraft", in which

the lewde dealing of witches and witchmongers is notablie detected, the knauerie of coniurors, the impietie of inchantors, the follie of soothsaiers, the impudent falshood of cousenors, the infidelitie of atheists, the pestilent practises of pythonists, the curiositie of figurecasters, the vanitie of dreamers, the beggerlie art of alcumystrie, the abhomination of idolatrie, the horrible art of poisoning.

Contrary to appearances Scot was not the Witch-finder General but rather a Justice of the Peace. He went on to show how the same effects that were thought to be caused by dabbling in the forbidden arts could be brought about by "the vertue and power of naturall magike". This was the first book in English to reveal the secrets of sleights of hand. He described the methods used by fairground jugglers when hiding and moving balls under cups, changing money and shuffling cards. As the seventeenth century progressed a succession of books rolled off the presses devoted solely to conjuring and to demonstrating that its wonders were accomplished by purely natural means. By the eighteenth century, with the help of the bright rays of the Enlightenment, people were able to view magic simply as a secular trick, a sleight of hand, even a sophisticated illusion.

Another less obvious influence on the art's increasing respectability was simply that of a change of venue. In the early seventeen hundreds most magicians were performing at fairs. However, during the second half of the century many fairs, which were increasingly being seen as a threat to local traders and to public morals, were shortened and scaled back by the authorities. (For example, in 1751 the outraged residents of Hull took to the streets when the town's traditional sixteen-day fair was cut by eleven days.) Many conjurors responded to this threat to their income by hiring venues in inns, public houses or assembly rooms and by making use of the growing network of small theatres for their shows.

As it turned out, taking their performances inside helped magicians to change the impression that conjuring was simply the preserve of street entertainers who were seeking to defraud the public. Instead of tricking people out of their money they now earned this money by entertaining people with their "deceptions". Gradually, this helped conjuring to become popular as a form of entertainment among all levels of society, including the upper classes. So, by the end of the seventeen hundreds, the most famous magicians were able to tour the capital cities of Europe, hiring and filling large theatres as they went.

Magicians also found their art and reputation being transformed by developments in the apparently unspectacular world of engineering. Performing in the 1720s, Isaac Fawkes was the greatest

British conjuror of the first half of the century and played a major role in legitimising the art, both here and abroad. In part this was through his use of mechanical devices that had been created for him by Christopher Pinchbeck, a genius of design and engineering. The most famous of these was used by Fawkes to perform the "Marvellous Flower Trick" in which a tree would grow out of a plant pot, blossom, and bear fruit that members of the audience could then eat. Through the second half of the century other magicians followed Fawkes's lead and used a wide range of increasingly sophisticated machinery. For example, the French conjuror Comus displayed such automata as "The Learned Mermaid" and a figure that put on clothes chosen by the spectators.

Along with these technological aids, magicians also began to make use of discoveries in science to help create or enhance their illusions. For example, after Brand's discovery of phosphorus in 1669, those in the entertainment industry exploited the ability of the Devil's Element to amaze. However, phosphorus did not come cheaply. Robert Boyle sold it for fifty shillings an ounce and, a century later, a book entitled "The Conjuror's Repository" warned that the substance was so expensive that few could afford to play many tricks with it at home.[7]

"The Conjuror's Repository, or the whole art and mystery of magic displayed" disclosed the deceptions of many "Celebrated Characters" including Katterfelto. Several of the tricks in the book involve phosphorus, such as how to light a candle without the help of fire. The secret lay in sticking a piece of phosphorus, no bigger than a pin's head, to the side of a glass and then touching it with the wick of a candle that had just been blown out. According to the author this was "the preparation Cromwell used to fire off his cannon withal, very amazing to behold."[8] So, in a variety of ways, the growing relationship with science and technology helped to enhance the view of magic as a secular form of entertainment in an enlightened world.

Two final pieces of the jigsaw in the development of magic in the late eighteenth century were peace in Europe and prosperity in Britain. With the end of the Seven Years War that had been ravaging much of mainland Europe, travelling conjurors were able, not only to perform before new audiences, but also to exchange ideas and techniques among themselves. In addition, with its growing consumer society Britain offered rich pickings for conjurors, who came one after another in rapid succession.

Among the first to arrive in London at the end of 1765 was Comus, who was the first French conjuror to gain an international reputation. Comus performed successfully on and off for several years in London where it was said that he acquired no less than £5000.[9] Another arrival from the continent was Philip Jonas who, although he was reputed to be an Italian, may well have been another German. Like Katterfelto's subtle change of name, Jonas's change of nationality was a sign that Italy was gaining a special kudos in the developing world of magic. This reputation was boosted by two real Italians, Giuseppe Pinetti and Giuseppe Balsamo.

Pinetti was one of the most famous magicians of the second half of the eighteenth century. Born around 1750, the son of a Tuscan innkeeper, he understood the importance of style. Wearing expensive costumes and travelling in a carriage pulled by four white horses, Pinetti was sometimes mistaken for a prince. In around 1780 he travelled to Prussia where, the story goes, the royal guards were so impressed by Pinetti's display that they saluted him. This was witnessed by the indignant King, who gave the pretender twenty-four hours to get out of the kingdom. By late 1783 he was performing in Paris where his fame grew further.

Here, though, he had a heated row with a lawyer and amateur conjuror, Henri de Cremps, possibly caused by Pinetti passing off as his own a trick that de Cremps had invented. De Cremps's revenge was to write a book entitled "The Conjuror Unmasked", which exposed Pinetti by providing "a complete solution to all his tricks".[10] Pinetti responded by publishing "Physical Amusements and Diverting Experiments", although this revealed only those secrets that would not prejudice his trade. (Another work bearing his name was "Pinetti's Last Legacy – or the Magical Cabinet Unlocked".[11]) By 1785, with all these books on sale in Britain, he was definitely the man of the moment.

Pinetti himself had arrived in London in September 1784. Performing in the Haymarket Theatre, his advertisements combined flamboyant showmanship, the skills of a conjuror, claims to being a master of natural philosophy, and the promotional skills of a prince of puff. The parallels to Katterfelto, who had left the capital just two months earlier, would have been obvious to the public and may not have helped Pinetti's cause. Pinetti was the first conjuror in Britain to perform in such a large theatre and his charges reflected this, rising to five shillings for a box, though this also paid for his "able and humorous interpreter".[12] However, all did not go according to plan in London and there was a strong feeling that his audience was not getting value for money, as was reported in the press:

> *On Tuesday evening Signor Pinetti's reputation received a considerable wound in the failure of two of his most capital manoeuvres, particularly that of firing a nail through a card, which he attempted twice and was unsuccessful. In consequence of the second disappointment he had the temerity to run up and fix the card to the back scene. The imposition was too palpable, and met with a general mark of disapprobation. He was so much dispirited at the event that at the end of his performance his interpreter came forward and told the audience that Pinetti was very unwell and did not know when he should perform again. Notwithstanding which, candour obliges us to acknowledge that several of his deceptions were truly pleasing and wonderful.[13]*

A further performance was scheduled for the 6th November but it was postponed. Although Pinetti did perform again in the New Year, he returned to the continent in early February. Katterfelto had worked the capital for getting on for four years. The great Pinetti lasted for just over four months.

The other Italian, Giuseppe Balsamo, rose from humble origins in Palermo to gain fame, and infamy, among the elite of Europe under the stage name: Count Alessandro di Medina Cagliostro. Cagliostro was a magician, alchemist, quack physician and Freemason. According to Casanova he was also a skilled forger. Cagliostro was chased out of Russia by Catherine the Great for being a dangerous influence. He was thrown into the Bastille in connection with the theft of Marie Antoinette's diamond necklace, although he was released after nine months for lack of evidence. When he arrived in Britain in July 1776 he advertised himself as an infallible guide to choosing lottery numbers (something that Katterfelto was also associated with).[14]

In London, Cagliostro promoted a course of medicines, purgatives, baths, sweating, starvation and a diet of roots, all of which he claimed would indefinitely prolong people's lives. His wife, who was in her twenties, was presented as being in her sixties, while Cagliostro himself claimed to be many hundreds of years old. He went on to promote his own "Egyptian Masonry" before getting himself arrested on charges of theft and witchcraft. Having been acquitted once again, he eventually returned to his own country where he was imprisoned by the Inquisition for heresy. He was sentenced to death, although the Pope commuted this to a life sentence. In the true spirit of the adventurer Cagliostro made an escape attempt but after five years in prison he died there in the 1790s.

It might seem that Cagliostro was on a one-man mission to undermine all the progress that magic had made over two centuries to establish itself as a respectable, honest and secular form of entertainment. However, his great popularity shows that the culture of the time was far from uniform. Although, in enlightened Britain conjurors would not face the mediaeval fate of those who were found to be in league with the devil, "superstition" was not always easily replaced by "reason". A book published in 1784 entitled "Breslaw's Last Legacy" still found it necessary to claim that

> *the knowledge which the book conveys will wipe away many ill-grounded notions which ignorant people have imbibed. Some imagine that many deceptions cannot be performed without the assistance of the gentleman of the cloven foot, long since distinguished by the appellation of Old Nick, from whence the original of this amusing science gained the name of the Black Art. Indeed, some ages back, when learning was confined to a few, self-interested and designing persons pretended to enchantment and to hold intelligence with supernatural beings.[15]*

Certainly, by the second half of the eighteenth century Rationalism had made great inroads into the popular psyche and yet alongside it was the emerging movement of Romanticism. In many ways this was a reaction against the seemingly cold, demystified world of the Rationalists. Newton's universe was a reasonable place, made by a reasonable God and understandable to reasonable people. However, not everyone found this vision of the world either attractive or accurate.

One key event, in the many strands that came together to shape the emergence of Romanticism, was the terrible earthquake that struck Lisbon in 1755. Many thousands were killed by the tremors and thousands more drowned in the great tidal wave which struck the city immediately afterwards. News of the disaster sent further shock waves around Europe. It confirmed the growing sense of many: that the world was a far less reasonable and predictable place than the Rationalists claimed. Preachers interpreted the events to their congregations as God's judgement on lax morality, while the Romantics - poets, artists and others - began to explore a vision of life in which there was still room for mystery, myth and magic. In the latter part of the century, the popular imagination was attracted by both cultural trends: by a growing desire for rational education and by a lingering, or rediscovered, fascination with the mysterious side of life.

Ironically, we can see the influence of Romanticism in the public's fascination with the sciences of the moment, such as optics, electricity and magnetism. All these were regarded as "occult": as sciences that opened up the hidden mysteries of the universe and of human nature. They leant themselves towards the spectacular, often creating a sense of awe and wonder, and they were associated with matters of health and healing. As such they were well suited to the needs of the travelling magical showmen, who made considerable use of them.

In addition, for all their embracing of science and technology, conjurors were often happy to play on the ambiguity in the popular mind by trading on magic's darker past. One piece of advice offered by a French magician to aspiring conjurors in the 1780s was: "Do not claim supernatural powers when performing to educated people."[16] Despite this advice, performers such as Cagliostro continued to hint at links to otherworldly powers, or at the very least to what we would call the psychic - much as they still do. Likewise, Comus conducted a second-sight performance and displayed an artificial hand which wrote down the thoughts of the spectators. In short, he claimed that "his operations are so surprisingly astonishing that they would appear supernatural in an age and a nation less instructed."[17]

There was also ambiguity in the public's attitude to conjurors themselves. Alongside the more successful performers, who benefited from magic's fashionable status, there were still many "sharpers" who worked the streets and used sleight of hand to part gullible members of the public from their hard-earned or inherited cash. (In London during the 1780s their numbers were sufficient to justify the existence of "The Society for the Detection of Swindlers".[18]) As a result, although some magicians might find themselves patronised by the nobility, they were rarely regarded as respectable characters and could still be ranked along with "vagrants". They never escaped what Houdini called "the odium of the conjuror".[19]

Katterfelto was no exception. He, too, was keen to be associated with magic as a polite form of entertainment, but saw that there was a clever and respectable way to make money from the tricks used by the fraudsters. He set about revealing various deceptions, "which is very necessary for every person to see as many Ladies and Gentlemen lose their fortunes by gaming, particularly in London."[20] In other words, rather than take money off people in the street, Katterfelto tried to attract the well-to-do to his performances where, for the price of a ticket, he would use the same tricks to show his audience how to avoid losing considerably more money from the swindlers. One supposedly satisfied customer responded by penning some lines concerning Katterfelto's "laudable Explanation of the various Arts made use of by Sharpers, to obtain illegal fortune at the expense of the credulous":

High o'er all mean device he proudly soars,
And hidden fraud ingeniously explores.
There are, of human race, a baleful set,
Who would of others, dark advantage get;
Who, lost to honour, gain illegal bread,
And draw destruction on their neighbour's head,
Whose fortunes, lands, and credit fall and prey,
To thieves disguis'd, and scoundrels of a day.
Ye, too unguarded sons of fortune's train,
Who strive to bite the biter, but in vain;
Who stake the sweat of your forefathers' brows,
Or dip the jointure of an injured spouse;
Here see the artful villainy explain'd,
The mystic traps by which their end is gain'd,
And O! the all-alluring gamester shun,
By whom youth, age and fortune are undone,
And sure applauses must be due by all
To him who finds the pit, then saves your fall.
Honest to live is Katterfelto's plan,
His aim that honour's due from man to man,
Who further strives will fail in each pursuit,
And late repentance be the only fruit.
While pleas'd we Katterfelto's lectures hear,
We'll stamp his lesson on the mind – BEWARE![21]

Of course, one of the fascinating things about magic is knowing just how it is done, and this disclosure of insider knowledge helped to establish Katterfelto's own credentials for honesty and integrity. It also chimed in with his sales pitch to the ladies and gentlemen of rank, and increased the "value for money" impression of his shows.

Katterfelto also contributed to and benefited from the enlightened view of magic in an age of scientifc and technological progress. He made use of many automata: inviting people to see his "Swan and Mermaid", his "little Dutchman", "St Peter opening the Door by Command",[22] "the Black Prince and some other Machinery of Clock Work of the late Cox's Museum".[23] The latter may have included

his Coach self-moving still;
His busy independent Mill,
Contrived with ease your corn to grind,
Unmov'd by water, spring or wind.[24]

He made considerable, and costly, use of phosphorus. Sometimes this was to provide light for his "lunar microscope", and sometimes it was for entertainment, enabling his "wonderful experiment with a candle and poker"[25] or firing off the guns on his model ship. Electricity and magnetism also featured heavily in his shows. Sometimes this was for the purposes of enlightening his audiences; sometimes for entertaining them. Usually it was a mixture of both, as we shall see.

However, Katterfelto also played on the ambiguity in popular culture and on its fascination with the supernatural. In fact, he went even further than some of his fellow performers by dropping strong hints that the seemingly inexplicable aspects of his magical performances were due to the influence of demonic powers. By doing so he gave himself further opportunities to entertain and amuse the public. A little hint of mystery, fascination and even danger was a good crowd-puller, then as now.

References to his "caprimantic art" had been around since his first adverts in York. However, it wasn't until 1783 that the darker side of Katterfelto's publicity really came to the fore. In the third year of his London run, and having exhausted the possibilities of the flu epidemic, Katterfelto was clearly aware that he needed a new hook in the psyche of the public - a new "wonder" to unleash on the world. What had worked last year was old hat. He needed to draw new people to his shows and if possible get previous customers to return. So it was that he introduced to the world his "famous Morocco Black Cat".

The association between cats, particularly black ones, and the Devil ran deep in the folk memories of many societies. Back in the twelfth century, William of Paris claimed that "according to the idolatrous practice of this age Satan is believed to appear in the form of a black cat ... and to demand kisses from his adherents: one abominable kiss, under the cat's tail".[26] This was a practice that heretical groups such as the Waldensians and the Cathari were accused of. Similar charges of venerating cats were laid against the Knights Templars in the fourteenth century. A common theme in witch trials was the claim that the accused women had been given power by their dark master to change into the form of a cat in order to gain access to their victims. In folklore this transformation could be accomplished nine times, possibly because of the cats' nine lives. As a result of these beliefs the Middle Ages saw not only witch hunts but cat hunts as well. Shrove Tuesday and Easter were favourite occasions for tracking down and burning black cats, especially any suspected of being the "familiars" through which witches exercised their powers.

So Katterfelto was tapping into a deep vein of mythology when he began to hint at a connection between his beloved cat and the powers of darkness. The cat had been part of his act in the past and often featured in a trick he called "the Two Towers",[27] but from now on she became a central part of his advertising strategy. In April 1783 it was announced that, of late, she had

so much excited the attention of the public, as to induce several Gentlemen to make bets respecting its TAIL, as by the wonderful skill of Katterfelto she in one moment appears with a big tail and the next without any, to the utter astonishment of the spectators.[28]

Such was the reaction, that Katterfelto claimed "several thousands of pounds [had] been lost in wagers on this incomprehensible subject".[29]

The disappearing and reappearing tail was actually a variation on an old sleight of hand (for example, thirty-five years earlier in Berlin, Tomaso Peladine had removed and restored the heads, rather than the tails, of birds). By using this trick to make some extra money from his audiences Katterfelto was stooping to the level of the sharpers; to "the artful villainy" that he had so righteously renounced on other occasions. Later on, he frequently claimed that the Black Cat had won him the enormous sum of £3000,[30] and he expressed confidence that by the end of his stay in the capital she would earn him ten times that amount.[31]

One way for her to do so appeared in an announcement that a solution had been found to the age-old quest of the alchemists. Whereas they had been searching for the Philosopher's Stone which would transmute base metals into gold:

> *Wonders! Wonders! and Wonders! are to be seen by Katterfelto and his Black Cat, worth £30,000, let out of the bag by the Philosopher himself, who has discovered a secret more valuable and astounding than the Philosopher's Stone, the art of extracting gold from the body of a cat.*[32]

The money-making possibilities only multiplied when, in the middle of May 1783, he was able to announce "Rare News" of an event that would give universal pleasure: namely that

> *his celebrated Black Cat, who has nine times more excellent properties than any nine cats among those nine-lived animals, was safely delivered of NINE kittens, seven of which are Black, and two are White.*[33]

As well as fortune, his "Morocco Black Cat" was bringing fame as well, especially in the royal courts of Europe, where several of the Kings and Princes had reportedly expressed a desire of having one of the breed of this most wonderful and surprising of creatures. With the happy news of nine new members of the family came a chance for royalty to acquire one for themselves. So grateful was Katterfelto to his feline companion for his growing fame and fortune that he frequently announced he was giving her a benefit night:

> *Such therefore being the high reputation of the said Cat, as to induce the Queen of France, and other foreign Potentates, to solicit Colonel Katterfelto's attendance at their Courts, he is indeed to give her a Benefit previous to their departure from this kingdom, and is sorry the time is so short that he cannot engage the Haymarket Theatre on this grand occasion.*[34]

In fact Katterfelto had no intention of leaving. He even joked that he had plans that would keep him in London for some time, confidently predicting that "he shall become Lord Mayor of London, which he thinks will be the case, as his cat is infinitely superior to Whittington's in every respect."[35]

3. Advertisement, 9th April 1783

**For the BENEFIT of Mr. KATTERFELTO's BLACK
CAT!**

AS many Ladies and Gentlemen, who had
tickets, and were difappointed in not feeing the Exhibition laft Monday Night for want of room, they are refpectfully informed, the fame will be performed THIS EVENING, and thofe tickets will admit them. And THIS DAY
will be exhibited, at No. 24, Piccadilly, a great variety of
wonderful Wonders, particularly Col. Katterfelto's SOLAR
MICROSCOPE, if the fun fhines at the ufual hours, and in the
Evening he will deliver a Lecture folely for the benefit and emolument of the famous BLACK CAT, which has of late fo much
excited the attention of the public, as to induce feveral Gentlemen to make bets refpecting its TAIL, as by the wonderful
fkill of KATTERFELTO, fhe in one moment appears with a
long Tail, and the next without any, to the utter aftonifhment
of the fpectators. He doubts not, but all Ladies and Gentlemen fond of the PUSSY race, will favor this wonderful
animal with their countenanance and fupport, the more efpecially as Col. Katterfelto has no doubt of returning the compliment, when he fhall become LORD MAYOR of LONDON,
which he thinks will be the cafe, as his Cat is infinitely fuperior to WHITTINGTON's in every refpect. And Colonel
Katterfelto affures the Ladies in particlar, that the reports of
his Black Cat being the DEVIL himfelf, are not true; this
Cat, though endued with fuch rare qualities, being as harmlefs, and inoffenfive, as the Colonel himfelf!
    The Exhibition on the SOLAR MICROSCOPE, is This
Day from Nine to Four.

Whittington's cat was not the only one to find itself compared to one of "the greatest natural curiosities ever imported into the Kingdom". Some were saying that it was "the identical cat about which Owen Glendower used to exercise the patience of Harry Hotspur"[36] (a reference to Shakespeare's Henry IV, Part 1).[37] However, the most obvious comparison was not to another cat but to an altogether more sinister creature. Having witnessed the amazing disappearing and reappearing tail, many of his audience strongly suspected "from certain philosophical insinuations that this famous black animal is no other than the Devil himself".[38] Although the Doctor was "very sorry to learn" that people thought this, from now on the connection would be hinted at almost constantly, while always being denied with the most sincere surprise:

> *Colonel Katterfelto assures the Ladies in particular, that the reports of his Black Cat being the Devil himself are not true; this Cat, though endued with such rare qualities, being as harmless and innocent as the Colonel himself!*[39]

Katterfelto was playing the rational-romantic mood for all it was worth, and giving it his own feline twist. As an accomplished showman and publicist, with a genius for re-inventing himself, Katterfelto knew the value of spinning a story and keeping it moving to retain the attention of the chattering classes. So, having magical knowledge that excelled "the original Magi",[40] he began putting it about that some people held that he himself was the Devil, "otherwise it were impossible that he could shew such extraordinary feats in dexterity of hand".[41] Despite his rebuttal of these claims, on the grounds that he was a truly "Divine and Moral Philosopher", he ensured that the "rumours" continued to spread. On the 10th June 1783 the London papers reported that "a letter from Paris" had announced Marie Antoinette's delight at having received the gift of one of Katterfelto's kittens. However, she was "much surprised that the kitten has no tail". At discovering this, His Royal Highness the Duke de Chartres declared that "if his name was Kater-Devil in place of Katterfelto it would be more suitable".[42]

In later years, according to Katterfelto, it was not so much royalty as "many of the lower class of people" who believed that demonic powers were at work in him or his black cats.[43] One of these was a clergyman for whom, even when it came to heavenly bodies, Katterfelto's powers were attributable to the powers of hell:

On Wednesday 9th inst. a Reverend Gentleman, having regaled himself of a cup of ale, at some distance from Grantham, on his return home, was alarmed with the meteor which fell on that evening; the gentleman being unable to account for so extraordinary phenomenon, charged the celebrated Doctor Katterfelto (who had just arrived, in order to exhibit some lectures on divine, moral philosophy) with having caused it; and under that idea applied to a gentleman high in office for proper officer to conduct and send the doctor out of town, alleging that in case of refusal he should expect to have the church blown up and the whole town in a short time in flames; but his request not being granted, the doctor exhibited to the admiration of a numerous audience, and thereby obliterated every suspicion of the destructive power.[44]

A similar linking of magic and natural phenomena appeared in the Chester Chronicle following a storm: "Such is the potency of the *great* Doctor Katterfelto's *magic* that many continue to charge him with having raised the late winds."[45] On other occasions the list of candidates for the post of devil-incarnate included not just the sorcerer or his black cat but also his black servants[46] and members of his family.[47]

It didn't take long for others to pick up on this latest line in publicity. March 1783 saw not only the publication of the "The Quacks" print, with the devil standing at Katterfelto's rear, but also an engraving entitled "The Wonderful, most Wonderful Dr. Kat-he-felt-ho". In this, the philosopher is pictured "having packed up his Alls …trudging away with his Family and all his little necessary Appendices to his own Dear Country". With his solar microscope strapped to his back, he is making off with a bag full of "5000 English guineas", while saying "here be de Death of Philosophy and de Glory of Legerdemain". The implication is clear: he has deceived the gullible British public by substituting conjuring for true philosophy. Meanwhile his wife and three children look on, one of whom asks "Is my Daddy a devil, Mummy?" The cartoonist develops this demonic theme by portraying all three children and Mrs. Katterfelto with horns and cloven hooves.

Katterfelto responded quickly to these cartoons, declaring that "neither he nor his Black Cat bear any resemblance to Devils, as they are represented in the Print Shops."[48] Even so he must have been

4. The Wonderful most Wonderful Dr. Kate-he-felt-ho

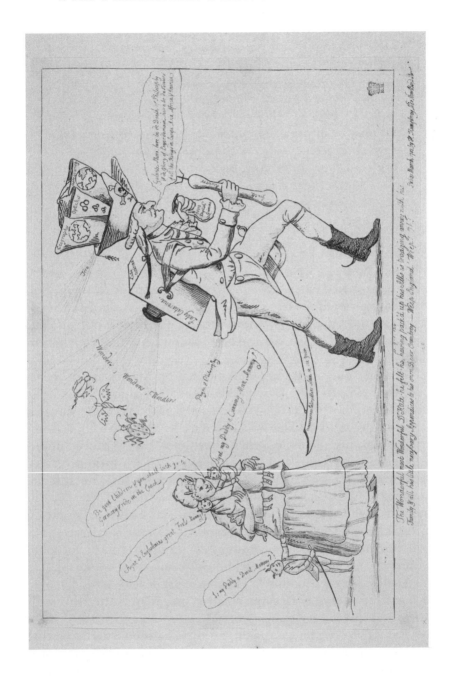

delighted at the amount of publicity that his own insinuations had created. This notoriety meant that, as with quackery, posterity would remember him for his "demonic" connections. In April 1792, the recently launched "Conjurors Magazine" received correspondence from a pseudonymous, and suggestively demonic, "Nick Katterfelto" (who was complaining that his answers to astrological questions had not been printed),[49] while as late as 1911 Roget's Thesaurus was quoting him as an example of a sorcerer, necromancer or warlock.

Given his devilishly successful marketing ploy, Katterfelto wasn't about to let the subject drop. In 1784, he reported a visit by our old friend the travelling Welshman (he who had fled from the army of insects), which led to "a very extraordinary affair" when

> one of the Gentlemen present asked the Doctor what he had done with his black cat and kittens; the Doctor, to the great surprize of the whole company, conveyed one of the kittens into the Welch Gentleman's waistcoat pocket at six yards distance, purposely to make that Gentleman believe he was the devil. On finding the kitten in his waistcoat pocket, the above Gentleman ran out of the room, and cried in the street, as well as in the exhibition room, that the diawel, the diawel, which is in English the devil, was in London, which caused a very great laughter to all the company, and that Gentleman has not been with his friends in town since that night.[50]

The Welshman and his astonished reaction followed Katterfelto around on his travels, as did various Gentleman farmers. At Derby in 1795 one farmer declared that

> he had laid a wager of one of his best cows that the Doctor could not make his watch stop.... The Doctor hearing this, requested him to produce his watch, caused it to stop going though at the distance of six yards from it, but shortly afterwards put it in motion again, to the great astonishment of its owner, who ran out of the room saying that he would never lay another cow as a wager, for he was sure that the Devil was now in Derby and all his imps.[51]

Another farmer at Whitehaven came to the same conclusion:

A farmer...seemed much surprised on entering the room, at the sight of the apparatus in view; and as his astonishment increased...he attracted the attention of several ladies and gentlemen then in company, who desired the Doctor to shew some of his surprising performances by feats of dexterity. From the smiles of the company, the farmer justly surmising he was to be the object of their laughter, cautiously clapped his hands on his breeches pockets, as a guard on his money and watch. The Doctor observing this and knowing that his credit was at stake, yet not withstanding the man's watching so carefully, in the course of five minutes conveyed both the watch and the money out of his pockets, though the Doctor was above six yards distance from the farmer, to the great approbation and amazement of the spectators and to the total confusion of the farmer, who, after recovering himself said that he was certain, from the care he had taken, no human art could deceive him and that either the Doctor, his Black Cat or his Black Boys must be Devils; however the farmer was not so superstitious but that he came again, along with part of his family ...and for fear of a similar disaster, very prudently left his watch and money at home.[52]

Conveying cats into pockets, money and watches out of them, as well as stopping and restarting these timepieces, were some of Katterfelto's favourite tricks.

Gun magic had been another staple of Katterfelto's repertoire since his arrival at Hull.[53] In 1781, he let it be known that "he will show the Art of Gunnery by firing at a glass bottle", which involved "making the ball drop into the bottle, or before it, without breaking the glass".[54] In later years others got in on the act, with his Gentleman Farmer helping to fire a pistol at "the marked Buttons and Rings in a Box with twelve divisions".[55] However, when it came to firing at a marked card, the best assistant and crack shot proved to be his own Black Cat:

One of our first Military Gentlemen...said, if the French could boast of having several regiments as good marksmen as the Doctor's Black Cat is (who, by firing several times at the five and three of clubs, at five yards distance, hit the centre every time) they could then say they had the best regiments of marksmen in Europe; but that fame the Doctor's Black Cats have only.[56]

Using guns in magic was by no means new. As far back as the 1580s a French magician called Coullew of Lorraine had been performing an illusion in which he caught a bullet in his hand that had been fired by his assistant. Although this sounded dangerous, in the end the real danger came off stage, when his assistant used the gun to club Coullew to death during an argument. Throughout the seventeen hundreds other performers developed different versions of the trick, of which one was Katterfelto's use of a bottle to catch the bullet. Given his track record for claiming things to be "new-invented" it is surprising that he never makes any such claims for this trick, nor in fact for any of the other deceptions he performed.

Instead it was another conjuror, Philip Astley, in his 1785 book "Natural Magic or Physical Amusements Revealed", who puffed that he had created the bullet catch back in 1762. Astley's colourful account is worth telling. He had been serving with the army in Germany and two of his comrades were set on fighting a duel with pistols. Acting as a second to one of them, and in collusion with his opposite number, Astley came up with a plan to avoid bloodshed. He inserted tin tubes into the barrels and it was into these that the bullets were dropped. Just as the weapons were being handed to the duellists the tubes were secretly withdrawn, along with the balls, so that only blank charges were fired. After his years of military service Astley started performing in Britain under the name of "the English Hussar", with an act that included a version of the bullet catch: "when he shall receive the ball on the point of a sword or knife." [57]

The development of the gun trick illustrates how, in the eighteenth century as now, one's fellow conjurors were at one and the same time rivals and a source of new tricks by which an act was kept fresh and exciting. In many of his advertisements Katterfelto refers to his own competitors in seemingly polite, even deferential, terms. For example:

> *After his Lecture he will also discover (gratis) all those deceptions that are now exhibited by Jonas, Comus, Boaz and Breslaw, likewise that optical performance called the Powers of Imagination, or Senses Deceived.* [58]

It almost seems as if he is giving credit where it was due, acknowledging others as the source of the tricks he performed, or accepting that others' names were better known than his own. Could this be a hint of modesty? After all, conjuring was an area of his show where he felt comfortable enough to allow his wife to take centre stage (with Londoners throughout 1783 learning that "Mr or Mrs Katterfelto will shew and discover several New Deceptions").[59]

However, we should not be misled. Katterfelto was revealing how his competitors did their tricks. Sometimes he did this for free: contrasting himself with his rivals who would "not divulge them for Five Hundred Guineas".[60] Sometimes he offered to do it for private audiences "on very low terms"[61] (which, in London, amounted to a full twenty guineas!)[62] As with his approach to sharpers, he was out to make money by disclosing the secrets of others. As it happens, this was a common practice among travelling magicians. For example, those who went to the theatre in Whitby in 1788 could see, between two farces, an act called "Conjuration Familiarized". This revealed the "modes of deceiving practised by JUGGLERS and SLIGHT-of-hand-MEN, in the various performances of BRESLAW, JONAS, KATTERFELTO, PINETTO etc."[63]

For Katterfelto, revealing how others did their tricks had a particular importance because he wanted to project an image of himself as a "moral and divine philosopher" rather than a common conjuror. To make the point he occasionally objected to being called a conjuror at all. Sometimes this was done by way of witty social comment:

Many sedate persons will have it that the Philosopher is a Conjuror...Doctor Katterfelto must inform the Public at large that, to his thinking, the best and real Conjurors are such that turn Bankrupt wilfully, and are not sent to Prison, and only pay two or three shillings in the Pound. Such great Conjurors are seen every day in the London and Country Papers.[64]

On another occasion he wrote that, having performed before royalty, ships' captains and many religious ladies and gentlemen, "he was never taken for a *conjuror* before he was at Kendal", where he had been incarcerated for his "new and uncommon experiments which some wise people call *juggling tricks*."[65] Sometimes he defended his status by criticising those who called themselves "philosophers" but in his opinion were nothing more than common conjurors: attacks that became fierce, even vitriolic. This was particularly clear when he crossed swords, or rather wands, with two rivals: Breslaw and Boaz.

Throughout the 1770s Philip Breslaw, a fellow German, had been performing in various taverns around London (as well as touring in the provinces each year, along with his musical "Italian Company"). He continued to perform in the capital through most, if not all, of the time that Katterfelto was in the city.[66] During this period there appears to have been no public animosity between the two conjurors. In fact, probably the only thing to cause Breslaw any concern was the Gentleman's Magazine's announcement of his own death in Brussels in November 1783. However, 1784 saw him remarkably alive and well. He was still in London and exhibiting exactly the same repertoire of tricks.[67] Soon afterwards he headed north, and in January 1788 the travels of Breslaw and Katterfelto brought them together once again, this time in Edinburgh. Here they both began to trade on the reputation of Giuseppe Pinetti - sowing the seeds of a bitter rivalry.

Despite Pinetti's relative failure in London, when Katterfelto and Breslaw arrived in Edinburgh, the Italian's name was still the one to be dropping. Breslaw had begun adding "Sieur Pinetti's Philosophical Experiments" to his act.[68] (Just how "philosophical" some of these "experiments" were is clear: "Several cards that the company may think of shall fly out of a Philosophical Bottle, through a little Shovel, one yard above the table.")[69] Katterfelto, too, was now performing exactly the same range of tricks, though as a "moral and divine philosopher" he was keen to make it clear that they were merely those feats "which Pinetti and other Conjurors call Philosophical Experiments."[70] He was also selling copies of "Pinetti's publication of all his various deceptions as exhibited in Paris" for 2s 6d.[71] All was quiet for a time between the two Germans, but once the magicians moved north, travelling up the east coast of Scotland, the atmosphere changed.

In August, when Katterfelto arrived in Aberdeen, he discovered that Breslaw had got there ahead of him and was stealing his thunder. To make matters worse Breslaw was preparing to move on towards Inverness - undermining Katterfelto's prospects for several weeks ahead. Once Breslaw had departed, Katterfelto, who proclaimed himself to the Aberdonians as a "Professor and Teacher of Natural Philosophy, Astronomy and Mathematics", thanked "all the Professors of the Colleges" for their support. Having established that the academic community was taking him seriously, he went on to declare:

He is very sorry to find that the public in general have lately been much imposed on by travelling conjurors, who have taken the title of Professor, when it is well known in France and in this kingdom, that Mr Comus, Jonas, Pinetti etc. never went by any other name than common slight of hand men, and perform most of their various deceptions by means of confederacy.[72]

However, arriving in Banff shortly afterwards and finding himself yet again hot on Breslaw's heels, Katterfelto lost his temper big time. He sent a letter to the Aberdeen Journal exposing the methods of those who performed Pinetti's tricks (which included himself, of course) clearly hoping that it would queer Breslaw's pitch with the public further up the coast:

On the 28th *August last, Doctor Katterfelto, Philosopher and Astronomer, was much surprised on that day, on hearing expressed by several gentlemen of that town, that a few nights ago they had seen all Pinetti's Philosophical Experiments by a Conjuror but with very little satisfaction to them. But Doctor Katterfelto expressed, if the Conjuror calls the Rings and Seals dancing in the Glass, and the Cards jumping out of the Wooden Bottle, and the Little Friar jumping out of the Pint Bottle, and Firing at the Fellow of the Burnt Card, if he calls them Philosophical, the Conjuror may well call them Experiments in Astronomy or Natural History, but Pinetti at Paris only calls them deceptions, as they are nothing else, and everyone of them are exhibited by the help of confederacy, which is behind the screen, which is made up in the room for the very purpose. The Rings etc. are fastened with a little silk; so are the cards that leap out of the wooden bottle, also the Little Friars; so the confederacy pulls the silk which goes through the screen to his or her hand, and that is called Philosophical by the Conjuror.*

And ... that card which is burned is fastened on a piece of board two feet long which is covered with two pieces of carpet of equal colour, and the one piece of carpet is pulled away by the confederacy behind the screen, and the card of the fellow that has been burned was fastened on the board before the pistol was fired, is called another Philosophical Experiment.

But if such a Conjuror was to come to the University of Oxford, Cambridge or Dublin, with such Philosophical

Experiments as above, the College Gentlemen at those Universities would make the Conjuror remember those Universities for a long time after, so that he would not come there again for many years.[73]

It was quite a tirade. Of course, the cost of preserving his reputation as a true philosopher was that he was limiting his own ability to perform the same tricks in that part of Scotland. His final jibe was also a little rich. Despite his previous claims to have exhibited "at most of the Colleges and Universities in the world"[74] and to have been heading off to lecture at both Oxford and Cambridge,[75] Katterfelto had always steered well clear of the universities.

If Katterfelto's attacks on Breslaw were focussed on the act itself, then his bitter row with Boaz was more personal. Little is known about the background of "Sieur Herman Boaz", though he claimed to have come from Paris.[76] In 1779-80 Boaz was exhibiting in the West Country and the West Midlands, and advertising in ways that were very similar to those of Katterfelto. He proclaimed that his

Grand Thaumaturgick Exhibition of PHILOSOPHICAL, MATHEMATICAL, STERGONIAGRAPHICAL, SYMPATHETICAL, SCIATERICONATICAL AND MAGICAL OPERATIONS …is of so striking and singular a Nature, as to be past all human Conception, and in an Age and Country less enlightened, would have appeared supernatural.[77]

Many thousands, including "some of the first Nobility and Gentry in the Kingdom", were flocking to see his exposition of the "Occult Sciences", which included his ability to

catch your secret Thoughts,
Whether your Virtues or your Faults,
And in an Instant Herman writes 'em;
'Ere you can speak 'em, he indites 'em![78]

However, not everyone was pleased to see Herman, particularly "Methodists and People of weak Minds" who, he said, imagined that he had dealings with demons. Whereas Katterfelto had claimed that such rumours arose from the brilliance of his deceptions, Boaz took a different tack. He played up the supernatural element of his abilities for all it was worth, although he claimed that his connections were of a more angelic nature:

> *He does not deny a Communication with Aerial Beings, of which the Learned know well enough that the middle Region of the Air is full, but this Communication he humbly conceives to be owing to his exemplary Life.*[79]

Thirteen years later, Boaz arrived in Birmingham once again, towards the end of Katterfelto's very successful stay in the city, which had lasted a whole year. Boaz's exhibition now included "occult and mysterious Operations in Arithomancy ... Phylacteria, Papyromancy, Dactiliomancy ... Palingenecia" and a "grand Meloskelothermick dish of Pancakes and hot roasted Leg of Mutton." [80] While challenging Katterfelto in his ambition to take the English language to new depths of obscurity, Boaz also took a pot at the amount of time that his rival had spent in the city, implying that it was time for him to make room for another. Katterfelto went ballistic:

> *The Doctor is much surprised that the Printer of a Newspaper, these fourteen days past, should please a common conjuror, by saying in a few lines of poor made verses the Doctor was a Prussian Rover, and had lived too long among the Birmingham Clover, which is more than any other Philosopher has done before...Such great Conjurors who pretend to have a superior knowledge and learning to all the different Professors of Colleges in Europe, by making Words which are neither Greek, Latin, Hebrew or English etc etc, but is only intended to humbug the learned and draw the ignorant by saying a New Hurlophusikon and Thaumaturgick Exhibition, and which was seen last Fair by many Servant Boys and Girls for one penny and two-pence each by other such conjurors, but as it is now exhibited at an Assembly Room, the brilliant Ladies and Gentlemen that are willing to be imposed upon must now pay two shillings each.*[81]

Katterfelto then set about demolishing Boaz's act. He claimed that Boaz must have thought that his audiences "have wooden heads to believe all that he sets forth of his miraculous performances".[82] The

"Meloskelothermick" hot roasted leg of mutton was declared to be an old trick of Breslaw's, in which the deck of cards revealed inside the meat had been placed there "an Hour or two" earlier. As for Boaz's magical pancakes, Katterfelto reported the great disappointment of those who "could not get a Pancake made in their Hats," while others were surprised "that the Farmers only bring Eggs to such Conjurors where there is Cards and live Birds in". Finally, he revealed the various ways in which Boaz's tricks depended on the use of confederates, who were often in short supply, "which is the real Cause why Humbuggers run from every large City or Town and cannot stay *so long in Clover.*"[83]

Having ridiculed Boaz's pompous advertisements, and having mocked his act, Katterfelto then began to get personal. Despite his foreign pretensions Boaz was actually "the Sieur from Newark upon Trent",[84] a "Penny Conjuror" and an impostor whose moral failings Katterfelto was happy to expose:

> *The Doctor could wish that Boaz – the Conjuror, who tells the poor Girls their Fortune for a Shilling, would take more notice of his Wife and Children who are now at Tinmouth near Newcastle, and send his present Lady to her favourite Farmer again at St Piese near Whitehaven; likewise that he will send some of his Pancakes and roasted Leg of Mutton that the Cards were in, to the Gaol-keeper at Northampton and some to the Keeper of the King's Bench, as the Doctor expects they will be glad to hear of Sir Boaz.*[85]

Katterfelto cannot have been blind to the many and great similarities between himself and Boaz: his style of advertising; the content of his shows; his allusions to the supernatural; his flattery of the public; and the unwanted attention of the law. This may be the reason why he attacked him so virulently. Had he recognised that here was someone who could seriously undermine his efforts to be treated not as a "mere conjuror" but as a truly great philosopher?

However, despite trying to distance himself from the ranks of his competitors, and despite attacking them and exposing their methods, Katterfelto never gave up performing his own stage illusions. Even at the height of his dispute with Breslaw in Aberdeen, he was selling copies of a book "published in London two years ago, expressing all those various feats in dexterity of hand that are now exhibited by Dr Katterfelto, Pinetti, Breslaw and all other conjurors that are now exhibiting in the kingdom."[86] Katterfelto would certainly have been gratified to know that, in later years, one of his customers reported that Katterfelto's magical skills were "very superior to Breslaw".[87]

These skills were an integral part of his act and blended seamlessly with his scientific lectures. In fact, for Katterfelto these visual wonders of the stage made an interesting comparison to the natural wonders that he revealed through his microscopes and telescope:

> *Here you shall see what is astonishing to see…optics and legerdemain, where you shall believe what you don't see and see what you don't believe – that Doctor Katterfelto is the greatest Philosopher and the cleverest Conjuror in the whole world.*[88]

As we have seen, the sort of fall-out between Katterfelto, Breslaw and Boaz was not uncommon in the magical "fraternity". All this was a long time before the advent of the Magic Circle in 1905, yet the need to protect the livelihoods of conjurors was already very evident: it was the need to protect them not so much from the general public as from each other! Katterfelto's part in this does not show him in his most attractive light, although given the fragility of his livelihood we can perhaps sympathise with his predicament, if not his methods. However, in 1783 something burst onto the scene that presented a far more dangerous threat to Katterfelto than any fellow magician or travelling philosopher. It would demand all his showman's instincts and art of puffing to survive.

[1] Houdini on Magic, op cit, page 57
[2] 6th June 1783, The General Advertiser, op cit
[3] 9th-13th November 1787, The Edinburgh Advertiser
[4] 7th July 1783, The Morning Post, 1st December 1798, The Newcastle Courant
[5] The Mirror of Literature, Amusement and Instruction, op cit
[6] The Encyclopaedia Britannica, 11th Edition, 1910–1911, vol. 6, page 943
[7] The Conjuror's Repository, op cit, page 118
[8] The Conjuror's Repository, op cit, page 112
[9] The Gentleman's Magazine, May 1766
[10] Quoted in Thomas Frost, op cit, chapter 7
[11] The book was being advertised in The Ipswich Journal during the spring of 1785
[12] 2nd November 1784, The Morning Post
[13] Quoted in David Devant, My Life in Magic, Hutchinson, 1931, page 165

[14] See the two items in Lyson's Collectanea volume 2 (2) p199 for June 25 1783, Dublin GP, and two in Sophia Banks, op cit, October 1788

[15] Quoted in Thomas Frost, op cit, chapter 7

[16] Henri de Cremps, quoted in David Devant, op cit, page 164

[17] Quoted in Thomas Frost, op cit, chapter 6

[18] 18th May 1781, The Morning Chronicle

[19] Houdini on Magic, op cit, page 58

[20] 11th December 1784, The Norfolk Chronicle, and 26th February 1782, The Morning Chronicle

[21] 28th August 1784, The Ipswich Journal

[22] 4th February 1793, Aris's Birmingham Gazette,

[23] 17th December 1795, The Derby Mercury

[24] 19th July 1782, The Morning Post

[25] 13th September 1793, The Shrewsbury Chronicle

[26] William of Paris, De Legibus, quoted in Harry E Wedeck, A Treasury of Witchcraft: A Sourcebook of the Magic Arts, Gramercy Books, 1961

[27] e.g. 3rd December 1795, The Derby Mercury

[28] 9th April 1783, The Morning Post

[29] 14th April 1783, The Morning Chronicle

[30] 5th April 1783, The General Advertiser, op cit

[31] 26th May 1783, The General Advertiser, op cit

[32] 6th June 1783, The General Advertiser, op cit

[33] 14th May 1783, The General Advertiser, op cit

[34] e.g. 9th April 1783, Morning Chronicle

[35] ibid

[36] 28th May 1783, The General Advertiser, op cit

[37] Act 3, Scene 1

[38] Quoted in The European Magazine, op cit

[39] 9th April 1783, The Morning Post

[40] August 8th 1782, The Morning Post

[41] Quoted in The European Magazine, op cit

[42] ibid

[43] 17th March 1790, The Cumberland Pacquet

[44] 17th February 1786, The Lincoln, Rutland and Stamford Mercury

[45] 21st January 1791, The Chester Chronicle

[46] 2nd July 1785, The Cambridge Chronicle

[47] 23rd January 1796, The Nottingham Journal

[48] 22nd April 1783, The Morning Post

[49] "Katterfelto" wrote once again in April 1792 in answer to other queries. Neither letter is printed.

[50] 19th January 1784, The General Advertiser, op cit

[51] 5th November 1795, Derby Mercury

[52] 17th February 1790, The Cumberland Pacquet

[53] 30th September 1776, The York Courant

[54] 12th April, The Morning Post

[55] 15th October 1792, Aris's Birmingham Gazette

[56] 27th February 1797, The York Courant

[57] 1st September 1777, Aris's Birmingham Gazette

[58] 22nd October 1795, The Derby Mercury

[59] e.g. 29th January 1783, The Morning Chronicle

[60] 3rd September 1794, The Hereford Journal

[61] 27th January 1790, The Cumberland Pacquet

[62] 6th April 1784, The Morning Post

[63] Theatre bill, 4th January 1788, Whitby Museum

[64] 20th February and 29th October 1792, Aris's Birmingham Gazette

[65] 26th May 1790, The Cumberland Pacquet

[66] e.g. March 1783, The Morning Post, and Thomas Frost, op cit, chapter 7

[67] 2nd November 1784, The Morning Post

[68] 7th January 1788, The Caledonian Mercury

[69] 18th August 1788, The Aberdeen Journal

[70] 12th August 1788, The Caledonian Mercury

[71] 5th, 12th, 17th January 1788, The Caledonian Mercury

[72] 25th August 1788, The Aberdeen Journal

[73] 8th September 1788, The Aberdeen Journal

[74] 16th April 1781, The Morning Post

[75] 20th January 1781, The Morning Chronicle; 8th May 1783 The General Advertiser, op cit

[76] Thomas Frost, op cit, chapter 6

[77] 19th April 1780, Aris's Birmingham Gazette

[78] 8th December 1779, Aris's Birmingham Gazette

[79] ibid

[80] 11th and 18th February 1793, Aris's Birmingham Gazette

[81] 18th February 1793, Aris's Birmingham Gazette

[82] 4th March 1793, Aris's Birmingham Gazette

[83] 25th February 1793, Aris's Birmingham Gazette

[84] 4th March 1793, Aris's Birmingham Gazette

[85] 11th March 1793, Aris's Birmingham Gazette

[86] 1st September 1788, The Aberdeen Journal

[87] The Mirror of Literature, Amusement and Instruction, op cit

[88] 6th June 1783, The General Advertiser, op cit

CHAPTER 5

THE INTREPID AERONAUT

*"[Katterfelto's] rhodomontade is very finely expressed in English
by the word puff, which in its literal sense, signifies a blowing,
or violent gust of wind, and in the metaphorical sense,
a boasting or bragging."*
Karl Philipp Moritz, "Travels in England in 1782"[1]

Truly historic days do not come along very often. A day that certainly
qualifies was the 21st November 1783. For the first time ever, a human
being left the surface of the earth and did not return to it for nearly
twenty-five minutes. In fact, it was two men, both of them French:
Jean-François Pilâtre de Rozier and François Laurent, the Marquis
d'Arlandes. Together they ascended from the Bois de Boulogne near
Paris in an air balloon made by the Montgolfier brothers, and in so
doing launched Europe into a new age. Almost overnight this new
wonder became all the rage and posed a grave threat to Katterfelto. He
responded with some of his most outrageous puffery. The early days
of ballooning involved tales of daring adventurers and Katterfelto set
out to place himself firmly at the centre of their story.

Of course the age of human flight did not come out of the blue. The
first glimmers of this new dawn had begun to appear twelve months
earlier. *Exactly* how is the stuff of legends. One story has it that, on an
evening at his home at Annonay in the south of France, Joseph
Montgolfier was watching ash ascend from a fire. As he did so he was
turning over in his mind the contemporary military problem of how an
army might capture Gibraltar, which seemed to be impregnable to an
assault by land or sea. In a eureka moment, he envisaged troops being
carried into the fortress by means of the same heated air that was lifting
the embers of the fire. Another tale has Madame Montgolfier hanging
a voluminous piece of her underwear over a stove to dry, only to find
it filling with hot air and rising to the ceiling where it remained until her
husband climbed on a table to rescue it.

Whatever the true inspiration, by the autumn of 1782 Joseph Montgolfier and his brother Étienne were making their first experiments in private. By the 4th June 1783 they were ready to go public, launching their first globe-shaped hot air balloon. This contained 28,000 cubic feet of air, weighed 225 kilograms and included 1800 buttons to hold together four separate pieces of cloth. After a ten-minute flight it landed some two kilometres away, only to catch fire and be destroyed, as a group of astonished and terrified peasants looked on. News of their success was sent to the Academy of Sciences in Paris where it caused tremendous excitement. After all, it was only two years since one of its most celebrated members, the engineer and physicist Charles Augustin de Coulomb, had confidently informed members of the Academy "that no endeavour by man to rise into the air can succeed, and only fools would attempt it."[2]

Before long, Étienne Montgolfier was in Paris collaborating with a man called Réveillon to make an even larger balloon. Réveillon was a wallpaper manufacturer and the balloon's appearance would certainly do his business no harm. It was a highly ornate affair: painted with blue and gold and bearing designs of the zodiac and the initials of King Louis XVI. It took off on the 19th September and, with it went the first passengers ever to be carried into the air. Launched on their ten minutes of fame were a sheep, a duck and a cockerel, which all landed safely, if perhaps a little traumatised, some three kilometres away.

So if animals could ascend into the atmosphere with no ill effects, the question was: could humans do the same? Pilâtre de Rozier, a bold and ambitious young physicist, was desperate to find out. Through October, first Étienne Montgolfier and then Pilâtre de Rozier made ascents in balloons that were still tethered to the ground, one of which reached a height of three hundred feet. However it wasn't until the following month that Pilâtre de Rozier and François Laurent managed to persuade Montgolfier to let them fly free. However, by now the king had misgivings. Feeling that it would be wrong to risk human lives unnecessarily in the venture, Louis XVI decided that two criminals under sentence of death should hazard the journey. Pilâtre de Rozier was outraged that the glory of his achievement would go to two criminals. So François Laurent used his aristocratic connections to get Marie Antoinette to work her wiles on the king, who eventually succumbed.

The day finally came on the 21st November; at 1.55pm the

balloon began its ascent in front of a large and anxious crowd. As one witness later recalled, "Never a deeper silence reigned on earth: admiration, terror, and pity could be read on all faces."[3] François Laurent waved his handkerchief to reassure the crowd below that all was well, which then erupted into cheers. Carried by the wind, the balloon was kept aloft by the handfuls of straw that the two adventurers used to stoke the fire. News of the flight spread rapidly and countless Parisians came out onto the streets or climbed buildings to get a better view. After a journey of ten kilometres the aeronauts landed beyond the city walls. Of all the risks involved in that momentous journey the greatest danger may have been the crowd of peasants and labourers who then besieged them, tearing Pilâtre de Rozier's overcoats into shreds for souvenirs. History had been made and they wanted a part of it.

The impact on the public in France can hardly be overestimated. Marie Antoinette declared ballooning to be "the sport of the gods", and "balloonmania" soon began to rage and spread rapidly across Europe and as far afield as North America. Within weeks, balloon launches were reported in Madrid, The Hague, Hamburg, Berlin, and Copenhagen. At first, however, the reaction in Britain was mixed. Some saw balloons as no more than a sophisticated toy, while Joseph Banks, President of the Royal Society, was sceptical of the scientific usefulness of ballooning. Behind some of the scepticism was a disappointment that the honour of first exploring the skies had gone to the old enemy and rival over the English Channel. The newspapers reflected these feelings, urging "all men to laugh this new folly out of practice as soon as possible."[4]

At first Katterfelto tapped into this negative assessment of the new phenomenon, although for a different reason. He knew that it could prove to be a great and mighty wonder, and a major rival for the attention of his customers. In the face of these new heroes of the air he was in danger of becoming yesterday's man, especially as he was now beginning his fourth year in the capital. So Katterfelto went onto the offensive. On the 6th December he swung his weight behind the anti-ballooning lobby, declaring to the world that he had invented something of far greater value to the world than a few balloons. It was his "alarum", his supposedly new method of creating light and fire, which he declared to be "more useful than 10,000 Air Balloons."[5] Just as the balloons grew bigger, so Katterfelto's hot air soon increased the superiority of his invention over its rivals:

Half a crown's worth of that valuable article in a house or ship is better sometimes than £5,000 or £10,000, as many lives may be saved by it, and is more useful to the public than 20,000 Air Balloons.[6]

Within a fortnight, this inflated to being better than £20,000 and 30,000 air balloons.[7] Katterfelto was not a prince of puff for nothing. However, the sceptics were not having it all their own way. In the autumn of 1783 a flurry of aerial launches began in London. Because of the widespread jealousy and jingoism, many of these pioneers of ballooning in Britain came from the continent. The first were two Italians: Michael Biaginni, an artificial flower seller, and Count Francesco Zambeccari, an exiled sailor and adventurer. Together they let off a small balloon in early November. On the same day as Pilâtre de Rozier and François Laurent were making history in France, Biaginni was announcing that another unmanned launch would soon be taking place at the Artillery Ground in Moorfields.[8] On the 26th of the month another pioneer, the Swiss scientist Aime Argaudi, demonstrated a balloon before the Royal Family at Windsor Castle. Clearly, despite its negative press, balloonmania was about to take off in Britain. Katterfelto realised this as well, and he knew that the best strategy was: if you can't beat 'em, join 'em.

He soon began displaying a fire balloon (a much smaller cousin of the hot air balloon) and offered to explain to his audiences how to make one costing "from 3s to £10".[9] (It was one of these fire balloons that had led to his arrest in Yorkshire when the farmer's hayrick had gone up in flames.) However, with the winds of change blowing ever stronger on public opinion, Katterfelto's new tack became clearer after Biaginni's launch at the Artillery Ground. Among the enormous crowd that gathered to witness the occasion, there was apparently someone who had seen it all before:

A Russian Officer, who was last Tuesday at the Artillery Ground, says he has seen an Air Balloon sent to the highest part of the atmosphere, in the year 1768 at Petersburgh, in honour of the Empress of Russia's birthday. It was made and let off by that great Philosopher Katterfelto; and was eight feet larger in diameter, but was out of sight in three minutes, and on a clearer day. The reason that balloon was out of sight so soon, the gentleman believes, is that the Philosopher was much better acquainted with the different inflammatory airs; and as that great man is at present in this metropolis, he could wish Doctor Katterfelto would make an air balloon of the same size and send at the same time his famous Black Cat, or one of his Black Devils up along with it.[10]

This is quite outrageous stuff. Katterfelto is claiming to have been the true pioneer of air balloons - a full fifteen years before the Montgolfier brothers. Like a magpie, Katterfelto was always on the look out for something bright and shiny that he could add to his show, such as a new scientific discovery or natural phenomenon. As an entertainer he always needed to have something fresh to attract his audiences. Sometimes though he not only says: "Come and see this fascinating new discovery", but also adds: "I thought of it first!" It is the well-worn strategy of many a childhood squabble, and it is most evident in his response to the advent of ballooning.

Not surprisingly, Katterfelto's puffs drew the attention of the satirists once again. In December 1783 an engraving was published in The Rambler Magazine, entitled "The New Mail Carriers, or Montgolfier and Katterfelto taking an airing in Balloons". The two men are facing-off against each other from their respective balloons. While being acclaimed by a person on the ground as "Wonderful! Wonderful!" Katterfelto is saying, in a direct reference to his boast, "Monsieur Montgolfier let us be reconciled." To this the Frenchman replies "Let us fly up to the Sun Mr Katterfelto", alluding to the ill-fated flight of Icarus and Daedalus and the dangerous folly of human attempts to fly. Atop Montgolfier's balloon sits the less than flattering image of a monkey playing a fiddle. Clearly the engraver is not just mocking Katterfelto but is reflecting the criticisms of ballooning as a whole. The two men are being watched by a crowd, who exclaim such things as "How soon can they get to heaven?" This question hints at a growing feeling, in some quarters, that the aeronauts were breaking free of the God-given ordering of creation. For some this was something to celebrate, as when one French poet wrote:

Infinite space separated us from the Heavens;
But, thanks to the Montgolfier, inspired by genius,
The eagle of Jupiter has lost its Empire,
And the weak mortal can draw nearer to the gods.[11]

For others this was a blasphemy; human beings had no business being up in the air. As another Frenchman put it:

Let us leave to each its domain,
God made the skies for the birds;
To the fishes, He gave the waters,
And to the humans, the Earth.
Let us cultivate it, my dear friends.[12]

In the "Mail Carriers" engraving, the flying demon, the "devilish" black cat and kittens on top of Katterfelto's balloon, and the comment of one of the crowd that "There's the Devil to pay in the Air", all make the satirist's meaning clear: no good would come of it all.

Despite Katterfelto's pretensions, the Montgolfier brothers, along with Pilâtre de Rozier and François Laurent, had gained a secure place in the annals of human endeavour. However, they only just made it. Hot on their heels was Jacques Alexandre César Charles, one of Paris's leading lecturers and physicists. Having heard of the Montgolfiers' unmanned launch at Annonay, Charles set out to build his own balloon. Not knowing what the Montgolfiers had used to fill their balloon, he decided to use "inflammable air". This gas had been discovered in 1766 by Henry Cavendish, although it had not yet gained its modern name of "hydrogen". It proved to be far more buoyant than the alternative, which was just heated air known as "rarified" or "montgolfier" air. On the 27th August, Charles's balloon was launched before a stunned and emotional crowd of Parisians. It rose to an amazing 3000 feet before descending forty-five minutes later in a village twenty kilometres to the north. Here the terrified villagers, believing it to be a monster, attacked it with flails and pitchforks and tore it to shreds. The public anxiety was so great that the French government had to announce that balloons were "only a machine, made of taffeta, or light canvas covered with paper, that cannot possibly cause any harm, and which will some day prove serviceable to the wants of society."[13]

Charles set about building a new balloon and on the 1st December, only ten days after Pilâtre de Rozier and François Laurent, he made his own ascent into the skies, together with a companion, Marie-Noël Robert. They took their places in a blue and gold gondola, toasted the crowd with champagne, and then the yellow and red striped balloon left the ground in front of what some have claimed was half the population of Paris. As it took off, one elderly lady in the crowd exclaimed in wonder and sadness: "They will eventually find the secret of eternal life. And by then I will be dead."[14]

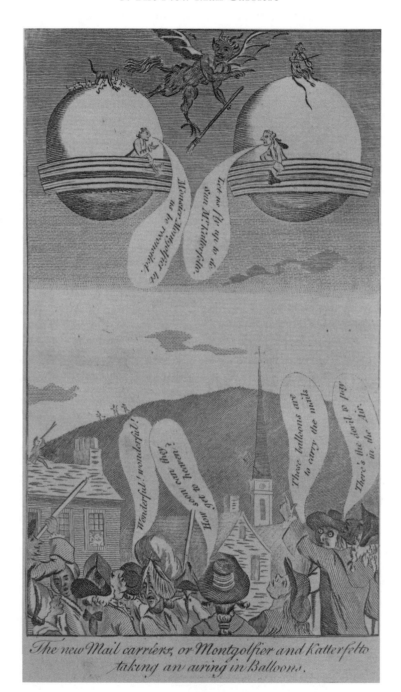

The new Mail carriers, or Montgolfier and Katterfelto taking an airing in Balloons.

Two new heroes were born and the hydrogen balloon soon became known as a "Charlière" or a "Robertine" in their honour. Balloon merchandising sprang up almost overnight. By mid-September toy hydrogen balloons were being let off in Paris and the French public could soon buy almost anything *"au ballon"*: there were bowls, buttons and beadwork; dresses, doorknobs and dinner services; fans, furniture and fillet steaks; pitchers, pots and puzzles; silverware, shaving mugs and snuff boxes; watches, waistcoats and walking sticks. You name it and someone was making it, in the style of, or decorated with, balloons.

By now, Britain was not far behind. In January 1784, a Mr. Clemson was offering to make Londoners their own balloons "to any diameter on the shortest notice and most reduced prices", which would be "filled with inflammable air ready for immediate experiment."[15] Merchandising began and popular culture soon got in on the act, with comic plays and musical pieces.[16] The craze soon spread out from London to the provinces. For example James Dinwiddie, the Scottish travelling lecturer, who had launched a balloon during December in London, was in the West Country in January launching one from Bath. It ended up in the parish of Farrington in rural Dorset:

It fell in a field among a parcel of cows who gathered round it hideous bellowing. The farmer and his men agreed to attack it, seeing it bounding on the ground, they concluded it to be some monster come to carry off the cattle.[17]

His next balloon fared a little better: being taken into military custody at Trowbridge where it had landed. Dinwiddie took his balloons down to Plymouth and then up the south coast as far as Portsmouth. Not surprisingly many of them ended up drifting out to sea, though one did manage to land safely over the water on the Isle of Wight. These sorts of losses added to the already considerable costs of launches. So as well as charging to view the ascents, the aeronauts also recouped their costs by putting their balloons on public display. For example, Montgolfier's Balloon was soon being exhibited before astonished audiences at the Lyceum in the Strand:

This brilliant and most magnificent spectacle is doubly overlaid with gold! Upon it beam with effulgent glory, constellations of stars and all the planets of our solar system –

and, in fine, the whole exhibits the appearance of a huge world
floating in the incomprehensible infinity of eternal space! [18]

As fascination with all things aerial gained ever more popularity in Britain, so ballooning began to dominate Katterfelto's advertising, even though he still wanted to remind the public that with him they would get far more for their money than a mere balloon:

That Grand Air Balloon which Dr Katterfelto made 16 years ago in Russia at St Petersburgh, will be fully explained, and instructions given on how to make and fill such a one, it being far superior to any one which has been seen in France or England, and was made for half the money, he being well acquainted with the different kinds of inflammable air and as there is some in all kinds of metals, the steel and iron filings is the worst for any Balloon, and is not the lightest; he will therefore show and explain which is the best mode, that every person may make a large Balloon for a small expense; and as seeing a Balloon is only one article, and filling it only one experiment, he will therefore show three hundred others besides.[19]

By "the different kinds of inflammable air" Katterfelto meant that the gas could be produced by pouring acid onto pieces of different metals, namely iron, zinc or tin, although what he didn't realise (as no one else did at the time) was that in each case the gas created was exactly the same.

Warming to his theme, Katterfelto went on to declare that his balloon, which had made the historic ascent in front of Catherine the Great, had travelled the extraordinary distance of over a hundred miles in three hours – far beyond the achievements of other subsequent launches.[20] However, the real competition in Britain was not so much to do with distances as with replicating the achievements of the French, and as 1784 progressed the race to launch someone into the British atmosphere intensified.

The day eventually arrived in August and the honour went to a Scotsman, John Tytler, who took to the skies above Edinburgh. However his rise to fame was not a smooth one. Several unsuccessful attempts led to a "vulgar prejudice" among those who ridiculed his scheme as "visionary and impracticable and a private folly".[21] One example of this prejudice was the sceptical musing of a poet, who imagined the day when Tytler at last rose from the ground, only to have his balloon burst by a flock of birds, plunging him down upon a church steeple:

And thou, great TYTLER, what dids't thou then do?
Didst not thou then thy fatal madness rue?
When being blown from the sharp steeple's top
Thou could'st not then thy airy voyage stop,
But flee'st direct into a deep horse pond,
Where now you very nearly had been drown'd.[22]

Rising above such scepticism, Tytler eventually overcame the technical problems afflicting his balloon. As always, the media was on hand to report the historic event. On the morning of the 25th August a brief flight at last showed "that the aerial schemes of the French may be realized in Great Britain."[23] Two days later, following an ascent to 350 feet, it was not only France that could boast of its aerial navigators but Scotland as well.[24] Back on *terra firma*, Tytler was overwhelmed by the congratulations of the spectators who were agog to know what it had felt like. He was glad to tell them that he had experienced no ill affects from his journey but rather that the sensation had been extremely agreeable.

Tytler had made history, but only just. On the 4th August a Frenchman, Chevalier de Moret, had attempted a launch in London but the balloon failed to inflate. The large crowd, who had paid for the privilege, were none too pleased at being cheated of their spectacle and so they rioted. Other launches floundered over the summer. John Sheldon had actually begun to make his ascent when his balloon caught fire and he narrowly escaped with his life. The same fate befell Allen Keegan's balloon in September; the event was satirised by Paul Sandby in a print, "The English Balloon", in which a gigantic backside is shown going up in fire and smoke.

The first person successfully to emulate Tytler in England, just three weeks after him, was Vincenzo Lunardi, who was destined to become the star of ballooning in Britain. Lunardi, who was Secretary to the Neapolitan Ambassador in London, was inspired by the daring aerial exploits taking place on the Continent. In the summer of 1784 he acquired a hydrogen balloon and basket, or "car" as it was often called. Copying the ideas of a French balloonist, Jean-Pierre Blanchard, Lunardi added a couple of wings and a pair of oars: the wings to help move the balloon from side to side and the oars to row downwards towards the ground. Neither adaptation had any serious chance of being effective, but they did make Lunardi's balloon immediately recognisable in Britain.

Reflecting on the experiences of Moret, Sheldon and Keegan, Lunardi realised the dangers of "explosions or tumults" and made his last will and testament. By 15th September he was ready for the launch at the Honourable Artillery Company's ground at Moorfields. The interest aroused by this event was extraordinary. A vast crowd of spectators had gathered, which was variously estimated at anything between 30,000 and 300,000 (the latter would have amounted to a third of London's population). They were joined by the Prince of Wales, while George III sat at the window of the Queen's chamber at St James's Palace ready to observe the event through a telescope. When all was prepared the brave explorer stepped into the basket. As the balloon left the ground and carried its passenger into the air, the crowd looked on anxiously. Indeed it was said that "never did a foreigner leave this land with so many prayers for his safe return."[25] The basket from which Lunardi now looked down on the crowd below was also occupied by a dog and a cat, and was equipped with everything necessary for this scientific adventure, including a barometer and stopwatch. There was even a celebratory bottle of wine to toast the occasion. The ascent went smoothly - apart from the fact that it soon became clear that, despite all his detailed preparations, Lunardi had forgotten one essential piece of equipment, namely a corkscrew:

> He was enabled, when at an altitude of four miles, to distinguish corn-fields from pasture lands, so clear was the vision. The accounts which stated that his clothes were covered with ice when he came down, and that his wine was twice frozen, prove to be erroneous. The mercury did not at any one time approach the freezing point, nor did he experience any greater degree of cold, than being induced barely to button his coat. While he was proceeding on his way, he felt himself dry, but found himself without a corkscrew; in this predicament he determined on breaking off the neck of his bottle, which he effected with the utmost ease, and applied the neck to the following experiment: he estimated by his barometer that he was full four miles in height, and throwing the neck towards the earth, found, by means of his stop-watch, it was four minutes and a half in falling. He was enabled by its glittering in the sun to see it distinctly till it hit the ground.[26]

The southerly wind carried Vincenzo and his animal companions northward into Hertfordshire. After some sixteen miles, with the cat suffering from the cold, the balloon made a momentary landing so that the cat could be unceremoniously ejected from the basket. Rising again, Lunardi finally landed safely at Ware, having travelled a total of twenty-five miles.

He returned to London in triumph through the rapturous crowds and was presented to the Prince of Wales in order to give an account of his exploits. Lunardi's success captured the imagination of the public. His flight was reported widely in the press; many prints of it were produced and sold by artists; a medal was struck to commemorate the event; and Samuel Wesley composed "A March for the Flight of the Air Balloon". You could buy Lunardi crockery, glassware, handkerchiefs, fans and clock faces. The fashion industry went into overdrive. Soon it was *de rigueur* for a lady to be seen in a balloon-shaped bonnet, wearing her voluminous Lunardi skirt with its balloon motifs, under which were concealed her Lunardi garters. Lunardi himself was made an honorary member of the Honourable Artillery Company, and the public flocked to see him and his balloon.[27] England knew that a star had been born.

By the time Tytler and Lunardi had made their first ascents, in the summer of 1784, Katterfelto had left London and was on the road again, working his way through East Anglia. Of course, as the *true* pioneer of this new and exciting age of human transport, Katterfelto realised that he would soon need to join the bold and select few who could claim to have explored the atmosphere. So, having equipped himself with a balloon, he planned to ascend from Norwich in the winter of 1784. However, on the anticipated day, his daring-do was somewhat lacking and his flight had to be called off:

The 23rd of December last was the day that Dr Katterfelto was to ascend in his large Air Balloon in this city, with his two little black boys, and various mathematical instruments etc to take some astronomical observations. The day was very clear for it, but rather too cold for him to continue a long time in the highest part of the atmosphere, so Dr Katterfelto, therefore, did not expect it was in his power on that day to make observations sufficient, so he was obliged to put off his ascending; as he made his calculation by his thermometer, that if he had ascended three miles only from the earth that day, the cold must at that distance have been nine times greater, and he was to remain a few hours in the evening in the highest part of the atmosphere, purposely for astronomical observation, he would therefore have felt the cold still more severe. His aerostatic globe was made in London by Dr Katterfelto's direction before he left the metropolis, and is made of the strongest and finest taffeta, with a very large gallery round it and is 144 feet in circumference. It will contain above 100 gallons of inflammable air, which he intends collecting from charcoal, being the very lightest and best gas for an Air Balloon. It is the largest that ever was made in England or France, and was lately sent to him from London to this city, and he will shew the above Balloon to every company who come to see his new-improved Solar Microscope exhibition.[28]

Unperturbed by his first failure, a week later he was writing that once again he was soon to ascend, together with his two black boys. However, with no flight yet accomplished and with his time at Norwich drawing to a close, because of a reported engagement to lecture at Cambridge University, he reassured the public that he would indeed ascend "on the first warm, clear day in this city, or at Cambridge"[29]

The much-awaited moment reportedly came to pass on the 13th March 1785 back in London. An account of the event comes to us in verse form, written by someone "On seeing Dr Katterfelto's Aerial Excursion … in the presence of the King, Queen and whole Royal Family before Buckingham House, London". The omens were good as day dawned. "Fair was the morn, with orient's blushes spread" and so the balloonist made his preparations. However as the morning wore on the weather deteriorated:

Now Katterfelto, for his daring flight prepare
Through, the vast, trackless regions of the air,
Arranging with peculiar care and skill
His apparatus, the MACHINE to fill;
The ingenious artist soon his task completes
And no obstruction in the PROCESS meets.
Now gentle gales to stormy blasts increase,
Black, threatening clouds, obscure the heav'ns fair face.
Upon the earth descends their watery stores,
Tremendous thunder thro' the welkin roars;
In the machine an aperture was rent.

But none of this could daunt our hero's spirit.

> *'Midst these disasters, Katterfelto undismay'd*
> *No signs of dread, or tim'rous fear betray'd.*
> *But in this scene of elemental strife,*
> *Th' intrepid AERONAUT dare risque his life,*
> *When in his splendid car we saw him rise,*
> *Filling each mind with wonder and surprise;*
> *Till by degrees he gain'd a point so high,*
> *That clouds conceal'd him from th' admiring eye;*

The crowd, quite unnecessarily, now became alarmed for the fate of this brave explorer of the skies.

> *Who breast but with anxiety did burn,*
> *Pant for his welfare, and his safe return?*
> *Fix'd with a wish the public taste to please,*
> *His cool and dauntless mind no danger sees;*
> *Now freed from prejudice, the adventurer's name*
> *Shall stand unsully'd in the lists of fame.[30]*

There was also a report of another ascent on the 19th May, in a "new-invented Night Air Balloon" (which would have been nothing more then a balloon ascending in the evening but Katterfelto as always was keen to show off his inventiveness):

> *Being a very clear night, it was in the Doctor's power to continue in the highest region from 7 o'clock in the evening till 11 o'clock at night, and was most part of that time in a direct line over Buckingham-House and Garden so the King, Queen and all the Royal Family had the advantage of seeing that great Philosopher in the highest part of the atmosphere to the greatest surprise and highest satisfaction of their Majesties. [31]*

The London papers at this time are remarkably (and suspiciously) silent, knowing nothing of Katterfelto's presence in the city. These accounts of his aerial successes only began to appear in July and August when Katterfelto was visiting King's Lynn and Northampton. The feeling that all this is mere puffery only increases as further promised ascents during 1785 fail to materialise. In the September he was travelling through Lincolnshire, announcing that he would soon ascend at Hull along with his "two little black boys". Then in November at Boston he declared that

> the spot where he is to ascend is fixed by him and his subscribers to be half way from Hull to Beverly, as there is now as many subscribers from Beverly as Hull. The day of Dr Katterfelto's ascending will be noticed at both towns by hand and posting bills, and in the York Papers. The balloon is 108 feet in circumference, and is made of the strongest, finest silk, and is painted red and white. The Doctor is to fill the balloon with air collected from charcoal, being a lighter air than that from steel filings, and not inflammable. It is expected that Hull and Beverly will be, the evening of his ascension, illuminated, and we doubt not but both towns will be so crowded, that hardly any beds will be had for money, as we find the whole country of York have a very great desire of seeing that more wonderful Philosopher."[32]

Although 1786 arrived, Katterfelto the aeronaut had still not arrived at Hull and seemed destined to remain earthbound. In fact, the disappointed residents of Lincoln learnt that

> we are very sorry to inform our readers that we find, since the Doctor has been up in the high regions in his new-invented night's air balloon, he has, from that time, never been in a good state of health, it is therefore expected that he will be more careful in that manner he ascends the next time.[33]

Apparently he had "received a violent cold by his last ascending at London" (which by now would have been nearly a year previously) but still remained hopeful that by the time he arrived at Hull, if his health had recovered, he would be able to ascend in his "new-invented" balloon.[34] Of course, catching colds was as nothing compared to the danger of drowning, and in the autumn of 1785, and again in the early months of 1786, the Lincolnshire press was happy to deny premature rumours of the balloonist's death:

> It has been reported in London, as well as in the country, that Dr Katterfelto, the great and noted philosopher, was drowned coming from Hull in his Balloon, over the Humber to Lincolnshire, but we are happy to inform our readers to the

contrary. The balloon with the boat that were found last week
at Middleton, was not his balloon.[35]

After all this procrastination it is perhaps not surprising to find that after Katterfelto eventually arrived at Hull in October 1786 he made no mention of balloons whatsoever.[36] By now the public's passion for all things aerial was beginning to subside and Katterfelto was able, no doubt wisely, to let the subject drop.

Just as the ballooning craze affected almost every part of society, so the factors that led to its demise came from many directions as well. It had always had its critics: it was useless; it was frivolous entertainment; and it was an enormous waste of money. These voices only increased as the dangers became ever more apparent. In the summer of 1785 the pioneer of human flight, Pilâtre de Rozier, and a companion, Pierre Romain, were both killed trying to cross the English Channel. (The feat had already been accomplished safely on the 7th January that year by a fellow Frenchman, Jean-Pierre Blanchard, and his American co-pilot, Dr. John Jeffries.)

Although having conceived the idea of a channel crossing in the previous autumn, Pilâtre de Rozier and Romain's ill-fated flight wasn't able to take off until June 1785. It did so in what was a new concept in ballooning. They used two separate balloons containing both hot air and hydrogen: a dangerous combination given that the fire for heating the rarified air was very near the balloon containing the inflammable air. Not long after the launch the inevitable happened: the hydrogen exploded and the balloon fell to the ground, claiming the world's first victims of an air crash.

Another problem was that if taking off was dangerous, not doing so could be even more risky. Such were the dangers of disappointed customers starting to riot, burn balloons or attack the balloonists, that many balloons took off even though they were only partly filled, and many balloonists fled for their lives. As Dr. Edward Jenner, who would later become famous as the inventor of the smallpox vaccine, wrote prior to inflating his own balloon: "Should it prove unwilling to mount and turn shy before a large assembly, don't you think I may make my escape under the cover of three or four dozen Squibs and Crackers?"[37] Given that as often as not launches failed, this posed a serious risk to public order. In addition, balloons catching fire on landing could damage property and risk lives. So before long some British magistrates, such as those in Gloucester, were banning air balloons.[38] (In Russia, Catherine the Great banned all balloon flights for the same reason.)

Another fear, more imagined than real, was that balloons posed a risk to national security in the almost continual succession of wars with France. In the spring of 1784 the Morning Herald printed an "Epigram on Air Balloons", which seemed to develop Joseph Montgolfier's daydreams about assaulting Gibraltar even further. Given the story of the Trojan Horse,

Why may not then an air balloon contain
A flight of Frenchmen from the Gallic plain?
Long have they tried in vain flat bottom'd boats,
And now in air the French invasion floats.

An engraving also appeared entitled "The Battle of the Balloons", showing English and French balloons filled with soldiers shooting at each other.[39] Nor were the British alone in seeing the military potential of the new form of transport. A French print from 1798 shows an invasion force of ships and balloons setting off from French shores, accompanied by an army advancing on Britain underground, through an early version of the Channel Tunnel.

The balloon was also a gift to satirists because of its associations with "hot air". For example, Hannibal Scratch, the pseudonym of satirical artist John Nicholson, produced an etching called "The Aerostatick Stage Balloon" (see cover illustration) in which a variety of well-known personalities are pictured sitting on galleries around a balloon. The political leaders Fox and North are both there, as is the Pope. On the bottom tier sit Dr. Graham with the Goddess of Health, and Katterfelto with his feline companion. "Great Katerdevil" (as the artist calls him) is looking through a telescope while holding a sheet of paper that proclaims "Wonders, Wonders, most Wonderful Wonders"; the cat is asking its master whether there are any mice in the moon. The balloon, fuelled by the passengers' collective froth and vanity, is about to be burst by a mischievous figure with a knife.

The satirists found many other vulgar and amusing uses for balloons. One use that suggested itself was as a means of disposing of the undesirable members of society, such as politicians. A contributor to the Kelso Chronicle, troubled by the recently formed political alliance of the Fox-North Government, offered the following thoughts:

Quite ready for launching – 'tis now my intention
To prove the vast use of this novel invention,
By dispatching some rogues whose names I'll not mention ...

From av'rice insatiate, from spleen or ambition,
Having form'd an unnatural, curs'd Coalition,
They kick'd the State Ball to the brink of perdition.
Fix them both to this aerostatic projection
And let the wind blow in whatever direction,
Cut the rope – up they go see they swim thro' the air!
So they never return, it matters not where...
The effects this ascension must surely produce,
Will prove the Balloon is of national use.[40]

Ironically, ballooning's popularity also suffered a serious puncture because of Vincenzo Lunardi. As with so many stars, his meteoric rise was followed by a dramatic fall. After leaving London in 1784, Lunardi travelled up to Scotland where he made numerous ascents. These flights involved considerable risks, as was exemplified by his fifth ascent from Edinburgh:

This was apparently the most dangerous voyage he had hitherto undertaken, and the result proved it to be so. He was seen, about two o'clock through a telescope, by a gentleman of this city, to reach the sea, two miles N.E. off Gullenness, to the west of Dunbar, and three boats near him. The gentleman's observation has been since confirmed by the arrival in town, today, of some fishermen who picked up Mr Lunardi. The account they give is, that he was floating in his car, about two miles from North Berwick, when they set off to his assistance ... but that he was dragged through the sea by his balloon at so great a rate that it was three quarters of an hour before they were up with him, when they found him up to the breast in water, and very much benumbed with cold. When they got up with him he was six miles from land. He informed them that if he had not observed they were fast gaining on him, he was determined to have cut away the balloon, and remained in his car till they came up, it being hung around with bladders and he himself having on a corn jacket, which would have kept him afloat for a considerable time.... When Mr Lunardi left the car and went into the boat, the balloon having thereby been eased of his weight, and not being properly secured, mounted with great rapidity, carrying along with it the car, Mr Lunardi's great coat, his hat and everything in it, he having nothing along with him but the clothes upon his back and his sword.[41]

Clearly no sensible aeronaut would take off near the sea without his corn jacket and inflated bladders. Equally no self-respecting aeronaut would be seen drowned without his sword on! An even greater disaster was waiting for Lunardi in Newcastle where he planned an ascent in September 1786. As the balloon was being filled with hydrogen a sudden burst of gas forced its way through the narrow neck of the balloon. The men holding onto the balloon were so alarmed at this that, thinking it was on fire, they let go. Whereupon tragedy struck:

Mr Ralph Heron, jun. of this town, who had twisted a rope ... round his hand and arm, was dragged up by it to the height of, it is supposed, five hundred feet, when the rope and netting being disengaged from the balloon he fell into the garden adjoining which occasioned his death in a few hours.[42]

Britain had now followed France in having had its own fatal casualty from air travel. Vincenzo was inconsolable at being, as the report in the Newcastle Courant made clear, "though innocently, the original cause of the unfortunate accident." Others were not so forgiving. The next edition carried a letter attacking Lunardi and his fellow aeronauts, on the grounds that "no one has any right to sacrifice or endanger the life, health or property of another" as a means of following a whim or pursuing financial gain.[43]

For a while the show still went on and, perhaps because of a voyeuristic fascination with the dangers, it still drew crowds (as in Leeds where the audience may have included a certain Prussian philosopher who had arrived in town two days before).[44] However, Lunardi's star was on the wane. Soon afterwards he returned to London where, instead of ballooning, he began experimenting with a device for saving lives at sea - perhaps inspired by his dunking in the Firth of Forth. Short of money, he is reported to have worked as an hotelier for a while before heading back to the Continent to continue his aerial adventures there.

In the end, once the novelty had worn off, the risks, dangers and costs of ballooning had become clearer, and the satirists had had their day, the bubble of British balloonmania simply burst. Not that it went away completely, and for Katterfelto it remained something to be returned to from time to time as one more string to his bow. The poem celebrating his ascent before the Royal Family was regularly reprinted, always written afresh by a resident of Carlisle,

Shrewsbury, Hereford, Derby or wherever he happened to be staying. Occasionally people opened the morning papers to read that the great Doctor would soon be going to London to ascend once again in his "new ROYAL AIR BALLOON, by Desire of some of the Royal Family!"[45] There continued to be doubters, against whom he defended himself with "letters, whereby he will shew that he did once go up in his Air Balloon, as several people did see; but that is some time ago."[46] There may also have been believers; it was just a shame that they never got to see the intrepid aeronaut get off the ground where *they* lived.

Nevertheless, Katterfelto had weathered the storm. He had outlasted the whirlwind craze and he was still in business. Ballooning had also given Katterfelto the opportunity to extend his reputation as an astronomer. Even before the age of human flight his discoveries had apparently already proved to be of great value. As he later told the residents of Norwich in 1785:

The London, Dublin, Edinburgh, Glasgow, Aberdeen, Oxford and Cambridge papers express that the philosophers and learned at the above cities have a very great desire of hearing from the Norwich, Bury and Ipswich papers, that Dr Katterfelto has ascended in his air-balloon in the city of Norwich, as the learned gentlemen in the above cities do expect that Dr Katterfelto will make some very useful discoveries in Astronomy etc. etc. Dr Katterfelto being by all accounts one of the first astronomers as well as philosophers in the three kingdoms, and as the observations which he made four years ago at Greenwich have caused since that time a great advantage to this kingdom, particularly to the navy.[47]

Once he had been freed from the limitations of making his observations from below the clouds, his night-time ascent outside Buckingham House had led to further "astronomical discoveries" which were awaiting publication.[48] Even more revelations concerning the heavens were to be expected when the much-delayed ascent at Hull took place.[49] By the end of the year, the still earthbound aeronaut was able to announce that the findings from his ascent before the Royal Family had

proved of very great benefit to our navigators and it is expected will in time benefit the whole world in general, and as no person in this kingdom, or abroad, have made any useful discoveries by the ascending in their various air balloons, besides that great and wonderful philosopher Doctor Katterfelto, the gentlemen belonging to the Admiralty, as well as the whole Royal Society, have made a report to the King, that a salary may be granted to the Doctor for his useful discoveries, and if it is only £300 a year, they think it is no more than he is worthy of.[50]

Such was the value of these additions to human knowledge that recognition was expected not only from His Majesty but from the great astronomer's own peers: "It is also reported that Dr Katterfelto is to be admitted at the next meeting *a member of the Royal Society.*" [51]

Established in 1660, the Royal Society was home to all those who had a deep interest in knowledge of the natural world. It elected into its ranks dukes and judges, admirals and bishops, medics and Oxbridge academics, landed gentlemen and men of humble birth. Needless to say, with its motto, *Nullius in verba* – "Take nobody's word for anything" – it found no place for a travelling Prussian balloonist-cum-astronomer, no matter how vigorously he puffed. Yet this didn't prevent Katterfelto from styling himself from now on as "F.R.S.".[52] He knew just what he was doing. The most illustrious Fellow of the Royal Society had been Sir Isaac Newton, and it was on rivalling the great man himself that Katterfelto had set his sights.

[1] op cit, page 61
[2] The Balloon Era, Rénald Fortier, Photo Essays, Canadian Aviation Museum, 2004, page 3,
www.aviation.technomuses.ca/pdf/Ballons_e.pdf
[3] The Balloon Era, op cit, page 9
[4] 27th December 1783, The Morning Herald
[5] 6th December 1783, The General Advertiser, op cit
[6] 12th December 1783, The Morning Post
[7] 24th December 1783, The Morning Post
[8] 21st November 1783, The Morning Post
[9] 3rd December 1783, The General Advertiser, op cit
[10] 29th November 1783, The General Advertiser, op cit
[11] The Balloon Era, op cit, page 20
[12] The Balloon Era, op cit, page 21
[13] The Aeronauts, LTC Rolt, Longmans, London, 1966, page 36

[14] The Balloon Era, op cit, page 13
[15] 31st January 1784, The Morning Post
[16] 20th August 1784, The Morning Post
[17] A letter by William Ball of Shaftesbury, quoted in article for Dinwiddie in The Oxford Dictionary of National Biography
[18] 6th February 1784, The Morning Post
[19] 18th February 1784, The Morning Post
[20] 15th March 1784, The General Advertiser, op cit
[21] 28th August 1784, The Edinburgh Evening Courant
[22] 25th August 1784, The Caledonian Mercury
[23] 25th August 1784, The Edinburgh Evening Courant
[24] 28th August 1786, The Caledonian Mercury
[25] Quoted in article for Lunardi in The Dictionary of National Biography, volume 34, 1893
[26] 25th September 1784, The Ipswich Journal
[27] 22nd October 1784, The Morning Post
[28] 2nd January 1785, The Norfolk Chronicle
[29] 15th January 1785, The Norfolk Chronicle
[30] 20th August 1785, The Cambridge Chronicle
[31] 2nd July 1785, The Cambridge Chronicle
[32] 25th November 1785, The Lincoln, Rutland and Stamford Mercury
[33] 20th January 1786, The Lincoln, Rutland and Stamford Mercury
[34] 10th February 1786, The Lincoln, Rutland and Stamford Mercury
[35] 30th September 1785, 10th February 1786, The Lincoln, Rutland and Stamford Mercury
[36] 17th October 1786, The York Courant
[37] The Letters of Edward Jenner, John Hopkins University Press, c1983, page 3
[38] 18th October 1784, The Gloucester Journal
[39] Sophia Banks, A Collection of Broadsides, The British Library
[40] 5th March 1784, The Kelso Chronicle
[41] 30th December 1785, The Lincoln, Rutland and Stamford Mercury
[42] 23rd September 1786, The Newcastle Courant
[43] 30th September 1786, The Newcastle Courant
[44] i.e. 9th and 11th December 1786, see The Leeds Intelligencer for 12th December
[45] 20th January 1790, The Cumberland Pacquet
[46] 13th May 1790, The Cumberland Pacquet
[47] 8th January 1785, The Norfolk Chronicle
[48] 2nd July 1785, The Cambridge Chronicle
[49] 30th September 1785, The Lincoln, Rutland and Stamford Mercury
[50] 30th December 1785, The Lincoln, Rutland and Stamford Mercury
[51] ibid
[52] e.g. 12th December 1786, The York Courant, 12th May 1787, The Newcastle Courant

CHAPTER 6

A SECOND ISAAC NEWTON

*"He chanced to hear Katerfelto spoken of as a cunning man,
for whom there were no secrets in this world or the next."
G.J. Whyte-Melville, "Katerfelto", 1875[1]*

From start to finish Katterfelto presented himself as a "moral and divine philosopher". However, his philosophical and scientific lectures were always blended with showmanship. He lectured on optics and the eye, and then went on to amaze his audiences with his visual and microscopic wonders. He demonstrated "Experiments in Chymistry and Phosphorus"[2] and then created astonishment with the "magical" potential of the devil's element. He revealed the mysteries of "fixed and inflammable Air"[3] (i.e. carbon dioxide and hydrogen) and then amused people with the launch of a fire balloon. In the same way he combined many other spheres of knowledge and entertainment.

Magnetism was ripe for dual exploitation by Katterfelto the philosopher-showman. He lectured regularly on magnetism and the iron rich ore called loadstone and what better way to illustrate the lecture than by a demonstration of his magnet's awesome power:

By his new Discoveries the Doctor has lately gained so much Power with his large Magnet, as enabled him ... to suspend in the Air, all at one Time, four Pigs and four of his favourite Cats; and we hear that the Doctor is in great hopes he will shortly gain as much more Power with his Magnet, and suspend the largest Giant in the three Kingdoms in the Air. The Doctor has likewise a Load-stone of above 49ᵗʰ weight, which has been of great Advantage to him in many different Experiments, particularly in Iron and Steel Works at Wolverhampton and its Neighbourhood.[4]

Cats, kittens and pigs found themselves suspended "like a man in a balloon"[5] in all the towns and cities along Katterfelto's route from 1791 onwards. The giant never seems to have made it off the ground. However, in later years eyewitnesses reported that Katterfelto's shows in Whitby included his daughter being magnetically raised up, by means of a metal helmet fixed in position using heavy leather straps under her arms.[6] Pigs might fly and so might daughters but, given the relatively limited power of magnets at the time, it seems likely that these feats depended as much on Katterfelto's powers as an illusionist as they did on the unsurpassed power of his loadstone. Similarly, when he used a magnet to draw "the guts from your watch"[7] this may well have been a bit of clever misdirection to cover up an earlier sleight of hand.

As with other aspects of his shows, Katterfelto was quick to exploit the marketing opportunities presented by the public's attraction to magnetism. Along with his other merchandise he sold magnets of varying sizes for a shilling to a guinea.[8] Alternatively, if people preferred he would help them to create valuable magnets of their own:

> The Doctor is sure that his large loadstone will be of many thousand pound advantage (to Sheffield in particular) if he magnetises Ladies' and Gentlemen's knives from it, as he will explain to them that each knife after is worth above 100 Guineas at some particular times and for different purposes.[9]

Although mixing education and entertainment was Katterfelto's bread and butter, it did have its dangers when it came to being accepted as a great philosopher. Sometimes the fun got in the way of the learning, for as one witness recalled,

> though much knowledge might be gained from his lecture, people seemed more inclined to laugh than to learn; perhaps from his peculiar manner, and partly from his introducing something ludicrous, as on exhibiting the powers of a magnet, by lifting a large box, he observed it was not empty, and on opening the lid, five or six black cats put up their heads, which he instantly put down, saying, "it is not your hour yet." Also when about to prove the truth of what he advanced, by experiment, he had a strange way of calling your attention by saying, "But then look here," raising his voice loud at the word "here."[10]

Despite the dangers, Katterfelto persevered in his dual-purpose strategy. One perennial favourite was electricity. In 1782 the travelling Pastor Moritz observed with barely concealed disdain: "Electricity happens at present to be the puppet-show of the English. Whoever at all understands electricity is sure of being noticed and successful. This a certain Mr Katterfelto experiences."[11] He was not the only one. The great public fascination with all things electrical was a gift to lecturer-showmen throughout the seventeen hundreds.

Things had been moving fast in the world of static electricity during this period. It was now possible to generate and store large amounts of electricity so that it could be used to instruct, amaze and amuse. Two pieces of equipment were essential for this: the electrical machine, which had been invented in the mid-sixteen hundreds, and the Leyden jar, which began life in 1745. The first of these used friction on a rotating glass globe to generate static electricity. This could then be stored and even transported in a Leyden jar, which was a glass flask partially filled with water. The linkage between the two pieces of equipment was made possible by the discovery that electricity could be conducted by a wide variety of everyday things. This had been shown in 1729 by Stephen Gray, who had taken a boy from a charity school, hung him up by silken threads, charged him with electricity and then got him to place his hand over a plate of feathers, which all lifted up towards him. This experiment caused so much amazement that, before long, boys all over Europe found themselves hanging from ceilings.

The ability of electricity to attract and repel, to be visible as a glow emanating from the electrical machine, and to pass from one thing to another as a spark, meant that it provided a tremendous spectacle, which natural philosophers were quite happy to exploit. For example, in the presence of the King of France, the Abbé Nolle passed a charge through a hundred and eighty soldiers at the same time. He also electrified a whole community of Carthusian monks, joined by pieces of wire, across a distance of about a mile. Others used it to do such things as setting glasses of brandy alight with a sword and passing a truly electrifying kiss between people.

There was something truly wonderful about this new mysterious phenomenon. Imagine, in a world before gas lamps, being in a darkened room lit only by candles and a flickering log fire, and seeing something that must have seemed almost unearthly - the glow of an electrical machine reaching out into the darkness:

A Gentleman of the Faculty ... to his great surprise beheld the Electrical Fire ...above eight feet distance from the Doctor's Machine that he could tell what o'clock it was by his watch.[12]

Even more awesome would have been the blue sparks passing, like liquid fire, through the air between Katterfelto and his apprentice:

The subtle aether, which surrounds our frame,
Is by your lecture prov'd a liquid flame.
Your wond'rous engine, by electric friction,
Confirms the same, beyond all contradiction.
The azure fire, which you from it extract,
And by that fire the Wonders you transact ...
Attraction and repulsion, too, explain:
By threads, hairs, feathers, and a brazen chain.
The boy electrify'd, we much admire,
Who by his fingers give the spirits fire;
And from whose coat, hand, nose and tongue, we see
A flame ensue, on being touched by thee.[13]

The "liquid flame" of electricity was believed to consist of two types of fluid: "vitreous" electricity, which was generated by rubbing the glass ball of an electric machine and "resinous" electricity, which was created by rubbing such things as resin, wax or, happily for Katterfelto, cats' fur. This enabled his feline assistants to play a role, not only on the stage of magic and mystery but also in the lecture theatre:

His Black Cat has given also such great éclat to all electrification, that by all accounts Black Cats now will be of greater value all over Europe than what they were before, particularly among the Doctors, as he has proved by his great Deceptions that a large Black Cat will answer the same purpose as the best Electrical Machine for all Experiments.[14]

Other animals, namely frogs, played an important part in understanding the mysteries of electricity. In the 1780s, the Italian physician and physicist Luigi Galvani discovered that electricity enabled the muscles of frogs to move. Since the time of Newton it had been thought by some that electricity, the "elemental fire", was what made matter alive. Now this belief seemed to have been confirmed. It was as if the muscles contained little Leyden jars bringing life and movement, even to a dead frog. It appeared that inside the bodies of animals and humans was a permanent source of what Galvani's followers called "animal electricity", which might be available for other uses. Katterfelto, for one, took up this new insight, offering to "prove by Experiments to the Company, that their Bodies are Electric Machines, and that every person may fill a Bottle full of Fire without having an Electric Machine in the House."[15]

Another great advance in electrical understanding had come through the work of Benjamin Franklin, the famous American scientist and statesman, who argued that electricity was not two fluids but just one, that could be either positively or negatively charged. Yet, even this great scientist was not averse to a bit of theatre. He is reputed to have held a dinner party on the banks of a river outside Philadelphia in which all the turkeys had been killed by electricity. His most famous experiment, in 1752, involved flying a kite in a storm. The lightning duly struck the kite and was conducted down the wire into a Leyden jar. This showed that lightning was electrical and that this natural form could be made use of in just the same way as man-made electricity.

All this meant that in the world of eighteenth century electricians Franklin's name was definitely the one to drop. So, when the Comte de Grasse was brought to London in 1782 (having been captured during the American War of Independence) it was reported that as well as knowing Katterfelto from the Seven Years War, he had also heard Dr. Franklin speak "very much in favour of Mr KATTERFELTO."[16] (At the time, Franklin was serving in Paris as the American ambassador.) When the Comte was allowed to go back to Paris it was announced that he had been able, in return, to give a full account of Katterfelto's lectures to Franklin. This "raised the curiosity of Doctor Franklin so much …that the Doctor is determined to remain in Paris until the arrival of that noted Philosopher, which is expected on the 5th April next."[17]

Warming to his theme Katterfelto announced that he had recently received a letter from Franklin,

wherein that great Philosopher has favoured him with a number of discoveries on Electricity which Dr Franklin expects will surprise all those who are acquainted with the above apparatus in London.[18]

As a result, Katterfelto announced that he would be able to demonstrate these new discoveries, which had supposedly never been seen in Britain before. Enriched by the insights of the likes of Galvani and Franklin, Katterfelto claimed that his lectures on the "elemental fire" contained more than two hundred experiments.[19] There was certainly sufficient subject matter, spectacle and public interest for these electrical lecture-shows to span the whole of his career.

The need to find vivid demonstrations to liven up lectures could also be satisfied by the air pump. This had been developed during the seventeenth century and by now was one of the standard pieces of equipment of the lecturer-showmen. In 1768, Joseph Wright's painting of "An Experiment on a Bird in the Air Pump" had shown a travelling scientist creating a vacuum in a glass flask containing a cockatoo. Katterfelto boasted of "an air pump so capable of refining the quantity of air, as to kill with its salubrity".[20] However, for reasons of cost and availability, sparrows rather than cockatoos would have been his normal bird of choice, kept in the cages that Robert Hird remembered hanging from the outside of Katterfelto's wagon in Bedale.[21] Hird also went on to tell how the Doctor's cats sometimes played a similar, though not fatal, role:

he did keep them to shew skill,
And shew the use of air,
Which he divested at his will,
As dead they did appear![22]

Katterfelto's lectures on the air pump went beyond spectacular demonstrations, although not everyone was impressed by the accuracy of the scientific understanding they contained. In 1787, the Newcastle Courant carried a review of one such lecture given at North Shields, which had been attended by a gentleman called Patrick Holland. Holland, finding that he disagreed with Katterfelto about the effects of high air pressure on human beings, began to heckle:

Last Friday I went with a friend to hear the pretending
Philosopher Katterfelto, whose lecture was to be either on
Electricity or Magnetism; but at my going he began with the
air pump, on which, he explained every part contrary to
reason, and more particularly in thick or clear weather, for he

makes man, in clear weather, that is, when the air is strong, to be so prest that he cannot move; and I find in close foggy weather, only, we are in that situation ... He and I had some words on the subject, but could not get one satisfactory answer from him, only ill-language.

Although this was a rather obscure argument, Holland went on to point out a clear flaw in Katterfelto's lecture when it came to the cause of the tides: Katterfelto had apparently explained the tides by saying that they were pressed by the moon rather than being attracted to it by the pull of gravity. As the evening wore on, Holland became increasingly frustrated and eventually challenged Katterfelto to the equivalent of a scientific duel:

And as his behaviour was very rude during his performance, as soon as he was done, I stept up to him, and offered to convince the public that he was an impostor. I begun with the tides, to which he would give me no reply, but offered to give me a meeting at nine o'clock next morning; at which time I went with a gentleman, but he would not come to a hearing on any matter. I offered to give him his choice in either natural or moral philosophy, with either mathematical or metaphysical demonstrations, which he refused, pretending that he only had a right to shew his instruments.

So I would have every gentleman who has a son to be aware of him, as he may infuse such principles into his head that the best authors will have enough to do to eradicate.

I am Gentlemen, Your humble Servant,
Patrick Holland[23]

We have seen enough of Katterfelto to know that he would be unlikely to take such an assault on his reputation lying down. Sure enough, a week later the newspaper carried his hostile and sarcastic reply:

Doctor Katterfelto, Experimental Philosopher, was much surprized that a very illiterate person, one Patrick Holland, Commander of a coal ship, has taken the liberty to injure his character; but as Doctor Katterfelto's merits are well known in London, as well as in the country, as he delivers his variety

*of Lectures, and shews the Experiments of Sir Isaac Newton
and other Philosophers' principles; he hopes, therefore, that the
advertisement has been very little noticed among the learned
… Patrick Holland paid only one shilling for a back seat, like
other servants, for one night. He, therefore, knows much of
Doctor Katterfelto's Lectures and Experiments; he also
exprest that Doctor Katterfelto was the first and last
Philosopher which he would see exhibit, but he will have it,
that no Gentleman at North Shields is able to converse with
him about Philosophy or any Science, but by all accounts,
which is well known in that town, Patrick Holland received
his great education at Morpeth, in a school where they pay 3d
or 6d a week.*

After this attack on his opponent's academic background, Katterfelto
suggested that Holland's lack of understanding about air pressure
had a gastronomic cause. From his school days until the present,
Holland had been eating far too much "crowdie" (a kind of soft
cheese) which had dulled his wits and made him think that all
philosophers who disagreed with him were impostors. Katterfelto
then concluded by ridiculing Holland's own pretensions to be a
natural philosopher:

*But Doctor Katterfelto thinks, if there is an imposter now in
the country, or a second bottle conjuror, Patrick Holland may
pass for one, as ten days ago he was to make a great explosion
at Tynemouth, and several of his friends went, and waited
over three hours to see his grand experiments, but he not
knowing the proper composition, the explosion is to be yet …
Doctor Katterfelto, therefore, thinks that Patrick Holland has
made himself a Barometer of crowdie, that the crowdie may
stand the highest degree in very cloudy days or nights, and
remain in the lowest degree in a clear day, or dry
atmosphere.*[24]

Clearly, Holland saw Katterfelto as more of a fraud than a
philosopher. However, perhaps wisely, he let the matter drop.

Katterfelto's assessment of himself was, of course, very different.
His various discoveries and inventions proclaimed him to be not
only a man of brilliance but also of immense worth. The challenge for
Katterfelto, shared by other eighteenth century natural philosophers,

was to show society that he could be of some use. Back in 1751 Samuel Johnson had expressed the sentiment of the practically minded British nation that "the public would suffer less present inconvenience from the banishment of philosophers than from the extinction of any common trade."[25] Rising to the challenge, as he always did, Katterfelto set out to demonstrate that he was "the most useful man in this kingdom".

With coal being such a vital part of Britain's fast moving industrial revolution he had plenty of knowledge to offer "all Masters of Coal-pits and different Miners"[26] in Leeds, Cumberland and Birmingham, that would be of great advantage to them. With the recurring threat of French invasion his lecture in fortification told, "How best to fortify and fence, Against proud Bourbon's vain pretence."[27] And with the challenges of navigation at sea Katterfelto could be of immense service to this maritime nation. From his days in London onwards, he repeatedly announced that certain new discoveries had received the approval and admiration of "the oldest Admirals".[28] Two of these were to do with magnetism, namely how to find "the North and South pole in cloudy days or nights without the help of sun, moon or stars or compass out at sea"[29] and also "the cause of needles' variation in different latitudes".[30] The ports of Britain learned that these discoveries would save both lives and money, to the tune of several thousands of each:

For the great benefit to King and Country and to all Mankind, particularly the owners of ships, and such that may go to sea from Liverpool, … Dr Katterfelto will this day, as he has the largest and strongest magnet and loadstone in the three Kingdoms, strengthen (gratis) all the compass needles for such ships owners and captains that see some of his days or nights experiments, which will be the cause that many ships, lives and property will be saved in one year's time, as it has been found by many navigators round the globe, the stronger the needles are, the more truer and better they make their voyages, and his strong and large magnet and loadstone is the only one in the three Kingdoms, and perhaps in all Europe now, that can do it. The Captains etc must bring their needles with them the time they come to see his days or nights Exhibition and they may have them again the second day.[31]

Or, as he put it in more poetic terms:

Ye who the floating ship advent'rous guide
First learn the important cause of wind and tide;
Learn well the compass-needle's varying power
And fewer ships Wild Ocean would devour.[32]

Other services to the navy included revealing the means of "letting off a cannon in a ship without fire; also of electrifying one hundred persons at sea without the assistance of a machine and to have water in a ship from twelve months and as fresh as at land". He was also able to show seafarers "how much time a watch gains or loses from the Sun in cloudy days or night".[33]

This last revelation sounds like Katterfelto's solution to the longitude problem. A ship's degree of longitude could be calculated if the precise time-difference from the Greenwich meridian was known. However, the clocks that were carried on board to show the time at Greenwich had always been notoriously unreliable. Katterfelto's answer to this problem seems to have been achieved with the help of his "sympathetical clocks". According to the ancient magical idea of "sympathy", an unseen connection between objects or creatures meant that what affected one thing could cause a similar affect on something else. In 1687 this had led to the bizarre suggestion that at noon each day an injured dog at Greenwich should be treated with a quack "powder of sympathy". This treatment was not painless and so would cause a similarly wounded dog on board a ship to yelp at the same time. By comparing this "Greenwich time" to local time the captain would then be able to work out his exact position at sea.[34] Katterfelto's clocks, supposedly "sympathetically" linked so that the chime of one caused the other to chime as well, would have had the same result. (Katterfelto could easily have created this effect on stage by a mechanical linkage or a hidden confederate, such as one of his servants.)

As for the matter of navigation and timekeeping at sea, Katterfelto had definitely missed the boat. This was the dawn of the age of "H-4", John Harrison's wonder clock. H-4 was so extraordinarily reliable that it enabled ships' captains such as James Cook to know their degree of longitude with an accuracy that had previously been unimaginable. Therefore, while many lives were indeed being saved on the ocean wave, this was due not to the Prussian Philosopher but to the achievements of John Harrison.

Unabashed, Katterfelto announced that his reputation had been carried far beyond these shores. According to "an Officer who lately arrived from Gibraltar", Katterfelto was regarded "in several parts of America" as one of the first Philosophers in Europe.[35] Actually this was to sell him short, given that "his Equal, by all Accounts, is not in the whole Universe."[36] Not to beat about the bush, no philosopher had excelled Katterfelto since the days of Sir Isaac Newton[37] and it was even possible that the great man himself had now met his match.

When Katterfelto floated the idea that he was to retire (offering to sell his equipment for £2500 to "a large school such as Harrow or Winchester"[38] or to a university)[39] the news was greeted with dismay:

> *If Dr Katterfelto, that great and most surprising philosopher, retires from his profession, as has been inserted in some of the evening papers, we may expect that the Arts, Sciences, Mathematicians, Navigators and the world in general, will sustain a great loss … Sir Isaac Newton himself, at his time, did not discover such various and useful knowledge as Dr Katterfelto has done these three years past.[40]*

Such was the pace of scientific progress and so fast were the secrets of nature revealing themselves to this "Star of Philosophy", that by the time he arrived in Sheffield in 1796 he was able to write that,

> *By all accounts this wonderful Philosopher has made more new Discoveries within these 12 years past, than all the other Philosophers in the three Kingdoms. Several learned Gentlemen say that he may justly be called the second Sir Isaac Newton.[41]*

Nor was Newton the only philosopher to find himself compared to the "Phenomenon of Genius":

> *When Plato his immortal precepts taught,*
> *And foreign lands Athenian learning sought,*
> *What admiration fill'd the assembl'd throng,*
> *Who caught the flowing periods of his tongue!*
> *So now behold, upon Edina's plains [i.e. Edinburgh]*
> *Another PHILOSOPHIC PLATO reigns,*
> *Before whose mystic, wonder working hand,*
> *Darkness dispels, and Ign'rance flies the lands;*

Fair Science opens her unexhausted store,
And bids her sons her greatest depths explore![42]

Over the years, Katterfelto announced more scientific breakthroughs in chemistry, optics, magnetism and electricity, all of which he expected would prove to be highly advantageous to Great Britain[43] and of greater benefit to the world even than those of Newton, his illustrious predecessor.[44]

He rested his case. Other travelling lecturers were said to have "yielded the palm" in acceptance of his greatness[45] and, in the opinion of several scholars from the University of Cambridge, Katterfelto was without doubt "the most useful man in this kingdom", who ought to be "taken notice of above any other person in the world".[46] His worth was also being recognised in his homeland where his Prussian Majesty had apparently commanded Dr. Katterfelto to send his many discoveries to the University of Halle.[47] (Here Katterfelto knew his stuff, as Halle was the largest and most prestigious of Prussia's universities, with a reputation for basing theology on the new science.)

If only, though, Katterfelto's usefulness to Britain was more readily acknowledged, then the nation would be both wiser and richer:

A Gentleman belonging to the Arts and Sciences, says he does believe if Mr Katterfelto was as much taken notice of in this city as Dr Franklin is at Paris, particularly in Court and in the Parliament-house, the public then might expect to hear all of more Wonders! Wonders! Wonders! Wonders! Wonders! and Wonders! of the Philosopher, than ever was heard of before.[48]

During Katterfelto's time in London he regularly expressed this hope: that his value to the nation would be recognised and rewarded by a modest salary from the king. In 1783 a figure of £40,000 a year was mentioned,[49] or, failing that, a lump sum of "£100,000 from every Sovereign" would not be too much.[50] (By comparison, earlier in the century Parliament had offered the person who could solve the longitude problem a mere £20,000: the equivalent of several millions today.)

Unfortunately for Katterfelto, but not for the exchequer, these appeals fell on deaf ears. However, the show must go on and in the summer of 1784, with his departure from the capital imminent, he was still pressing for royal and national recognition:

The only method of receiving information who has been, during four years, or is at present, the most useful man in this Kingdom, should be that his Majesty would be pleased to command, by the 11ᵗʰ July, all the Philosophers to assemble together at Westminster Abbey and to allow each an hour's deliberation, to make discovery of what knowledge he may be possessed of, that he may render himself of utility to his Majesty and the whole nation.[51]

Of all the "discoveries" and "inventions" that Katterfelto might have brought to this Elijah-like contest with the philosophers of Baal, few could have compared with one that he had announced in a blaze of publicity two months earlier:

This Day and To-Morrow, from 10-6 o'clock, there is to be seen what these 1000 years has been wished for by all the learned Ladies and Gentlemen – and that is the Perpetual Motion, for the discovery of which large premiums have been offered for many years past, particularly in Russia. It will therefore only be established in this city to the curious for a few days, as it will be sent to Petersburgh. It has been discovered through a long study by Doctor Katterfelto, Philosopher, and more than £3000 has been spent on that wonderful Motion before it could be completed.[52]

The search for perpetual motion was (and indeed still is) the search for a machine that keeps moving without the input of new energy. Katterfelto was quite right to date this search back a thousand years as the earliest known attempt was in Bavaria in the late seventh or early eighth century. The "magic wheel", as this device was known, was in fact powered by magnets placed around the rim, which were attracted in turn by another magnet fixed on the ground. This sophisticated arrangement could keep the wheel spinning on its axle for quite some time, although friction eventually brought it to a halt. Among those who had also attempted the feat was no less a mind than Leonardo da Vinci, who drew several machines that he hoped would succeed where others had failed. However, he seems to have been unconvinced by his own efforts and later drew a machine to show that perpetual motion was not possible.

It was the older da Vinci who was to be proved right. According to the laws of thermodynamics perpetual motion, or "free energy" as it is sometimes called, is an impossibility. However, this has not deterred many from pursuing the holy grail of energy production. Since the mid-nineteenth century when the laws were formulated, dozens, even hundreds, of people have claimed to have created such a machine. Far from dying out, the rate of such claims seems to have increased over time. As recently as 2006 a Turkish company claimed to have produced a free energy generator, which is supposed to work by using the "inertia property of material". The patent is still pending.[53]

In Katterfelto's time those who heralded the dawn of free energy were the showmen. Isaac Fawkes had advertised "a perpetual motion, where he makes a little ball to run continually which would last … for seven years together only by the word of command."[54] In February 1766 Comus had displayed "Perpetual Magnetic Motion" to Londoners, while Cox's Museum had contained another pretender known as Cox's Timepiece. This was a clock that he had developed in the 1760s together with Joseph Merlin, who also helped Cox to create his automata. The clock, which still exists today in the Victoria and Albert Museum, did not need winding and so Cox claimed that it was a perpetual motion machine. It could indeed run indefinitely but it also had an energy source, namely changes in atmospheric pressure which were transmitted to the winding mechanism by a barometer that contained a massive 150 pounds of mercury. As a result it failed the test of the "true" perpetual motion machine but to many it must have seemed to come pretty close.

Katterfelto's own version was, he tells us, an instant success. Overnight the whole conversation at Court, among scholars and the London public in general, became: "Have you seen Dr Katterfelto's Grand Perpetual Motion?"[55] Various Lords of the Admiralty, "Gentlemen of the Arts and Sciences", and the King, Queen and Royal Family (who supposedly had a private viewing of the new invention at Buckingham-house) were all reported to have been delighted by the wonderful machine.[56] By June 1784, Katterfelto was able to announce that he had taken some £900 in just nineteen days because of his new invention. Yet for all this attention the machine remained a mystery:

It is much to the honour of Dr Katterfelto, that not withstanding the many hundreds that go every day to see his Perpetual Motion, no one has yet been able to discover the cause of that motion; and therefore it will be an irreparable loss to the learned, whenever it is removed from this Kingdom. A few days ago four gentlemen arrived in London, who had come on purpose from Shetland to view the Perpetual Motion, and to find out its spring of motion, but without effect, so they returned home as wise as they had come. Likewise, last Saturday some gentlemen from the College of Dublin went to see it ... and returned equally ignorant of the occasion of its motion.[57]

Although this new wonder had been his final throw of the dice in London, Katterfelto continued to advertise it as he travelled around the country. For example, in Whitehaven his Grand Perpetual Motion could be viewed at any hour of the day, by groups of not less than twenty people, at the cost of one shilling each.[58]

And what was it that people were going out to see? It was actually something closely related to Cox's timepiece, in that it was operated by air pressure, though it served a different purpose. This becomes clear a few years later in Shrewsbury where he offered his audiences a chance to own one of these amazing pieces of equipment for themselves. They were able to buy

a new-invented HYGROMETER which may be truly called a Perpetual Motion, its action being continual Night and Day, according to the Degrees of Heat and Cold, Dryness and Moisture....They are prepared and sold for 2s 6d by him, and are about the size of a Pocket Watch.[59]

In Derby the hygrometer was revealed to have still further uses:

[It] will tell the change in the weather in a quarter of an hour's time, and will tell the dampness of a bed to travellers, and the proper heat to gardeners for a hot-house; and it also answers the same purpose as a Barometer and Thermometer.[60]

A hygrometer is, indeed, an instrument to measure humidity. Similar instruments were available, but Katterfelto was sure that his particular one would prove more useful to gardeners, farmers and travellers than the rival "weather glasses" which cost some "three or four pounds".[61] As if this wasn't enough, his hygrometer even turned out to offer a helping hand to the clockmakers of Sheffield by telling them the "the proper degree of heat to varnish Medals."[62] It was "the size of a watch to carry in the pocket"[63] and so, he concluded in the well-worn phrase, "no gentleman should be without one".[64]

In Wolverhampton, at the time of Katterfelto's visit, all this talk of perpetual motion stirred someone else to put pen to paper (with a good example of how social attitudes have changed since):

Perpetual Motion for to find,
Has long engag'd each studious mind, -
Long in suspense has hung:
Single – I said it could not be,
But – married – I too plainly see,
'Tis in a woman's tongue.[65]

As for Katterfelto, he was treading a fine line when he moved from exhibiting his instrument to selling something that could be "truly called a Perpetual Motion." In 1803, a Frenchman would be arrested in London for selling what he claimed to be perpetual motion machines. Katterfelto himself chose his words carefully and avoided saying that he was actually selling "the real thing", but he was sailing close to the wind.

This may have provided yet a further reason for his arrest at Shrewsbury. Once he was established there, he was soon taking the liberty of heading his advert "By Permission of the Right Worshipful the Mayor of Shrewsbury", and announcing the sale of his perpetual motion hygrometer. Could it be that the mayor took offence at someone making an apparently fraudulent sales pitch while using his own good name to help deceive the citizens of the town? (After all, it was the mayor who consigned Katterfelto to the House of Correction, even though the mayor was not normally responsible for the administering of justice.)[66]

It was not only travelling showmen who had to be wary of getting into trouble. In the 1790s travelling lecturers, and even scientists of the highest calibre, had to tread carefully as well. The revolutionary atmosphere in Europe and America meant that science had become charged with political overtones. Conservative thinkers such as Edmund Burke argued that science was politically dangerous. He attacked natural philosophers such as Joseph Priestley, a central figure in the British Enlightenment, who had argued that the new materialistic understanding of the natural order provided a model for reforming the social order as well. To Burke, these sorts of ideas not only challenged religious orthodoxy but also risked undermining the status quo and fermenting revolution. The task for the defenders of scientific progress was to show that reason was really a social, not an antisocial, force.

The French Revolution, at least before it descended into the guillotine-fed Terror, was supported by many in Britain, including Priestley and his friends in the Birmingham-based Lunar Society. Meeting at full moon, so that they didn't have to risk travelling home in the dark, the Lunars also included the steam-engine pioneers, James Watt and Matthew Boulton, Charles Darwin's grandfather Erasmus, who was a physician, and Josiah Wedgwood the potter. Many of them were Unitarians - a very liberal and rational group of religious dissenters - who were looked on with increasing suspicion as fears grew that a domino effect would lead to an uprising in Britain.

On the 14th July 1791, the streets of Birmingham were alive with the rumour that Priestley, who was also a Unitarian minister, was organising a meal to celebrate the second anniversary of the fall of the Bastille. A mob took to the streets chanting "Church and King" and "Damn Priestley" and over the next few days set about attacking Dissenting chapels and the homes of their prominent Birmingham members. One, William Hutton, not only had his house destroyed but his paper warehouses as well. To add insult to injury he was abducted by the rioters, taken to a pub where, having been forced to shake hands with a hundred of them, he had to buy them 329 gallons of beer.[67] As for Priestley, his home was left as a burnt shell. His claim for damages, published in the following February, reveals the scale of the devastation and the cost to his professional activity: £550 worth of philosophical, electrical, optical, mathematical and chemical apparatus had been destroyed; a library valued at £430; and piles of manuscripts, no doubt priceless in themselves but estimated at £420.[68] A lifetime's work had gone up in smoke.

When Katterfelto arrived in Birmingham in April 1792, the aftershocks of the riots were still being felt. So the possible political ramifications of his lectures were something that he had to bear in mind. In the past, being "a moral and divine philosopher", he had offered people his own thoughts on the social structure. As a resident alien, in an age when foreigners were often viewed with suspicion if not outright hostility, it was perhaps inevitable that Katterfelto's social philosophy was of a conservative variety. In London, although he never succeeded in his ambition to follow in Dick Whittington's footsteps, he had lectured on various "Celebrated

Characters in different Stations of Life": from "the Grand Signor to the Baker".[69] The rich man may have had his castle but the poor man at the gate had his own dignity, and so "Sweet Health and Peace attend the cottage swain, For which proud luxury may pant in vain."[70] Similarly, he advised

Ye mighty Monarchs, rulers of the earth,
Commanding dignity from royal birth,
Learn this important, serious, truth from me:
'Tis virtue only gains true dignity.
The Beggar who fair virtues path pursues
Shines forth as noble and as blest as you.[71]

In the turbulent setting of post-riot Birmingham this philosophy took centre stage. Despite being a foreigner he was a "Well-wisher to this King and Country" and began exhibiting "For the benefit to King and Country".[72] As such, he took it upon himself to fight the good fight against the Dissenters, whose own loyalty to crown and state was still a matter of controversy:

The greatest Liberty Doctor Katterfelto, the Prussian Philosopher, says a Tradesman or working Man can have is to follow any Trade that he likes, without having to Apprentice to the same Trade for seven years – which Liberty is in Great Britain and in no other Country in all Europe. An Englishman would think it is a great Hardship, if he could not go to a Town 10 or 20 miles distant to see his Friends without having a Passport, as they must have abroad. Farmers in this Country would likewise not be pleased, if they were obliged to go without Wagons and Carts to carry their Baggage 30 and 40 miles distant ... The people of this Country would also find it a very hard Case, if a Town the size of Wolverhampton or Dudley was lit up and their whole Property destroyed by Fire in a Night or Day's Time. And if the Inhabitants of Birmingham etc were to have 2, 5, 10 or more Soldiers House for House, quartered on them according to Size in War or no War Time ... the Doctor expects many persons would envy the Old Liberty again. And it is well known that the late King of Prussia left all the Money to the Nation, as other Kings must do when they die. A King or Lord does not carry much more out of this World than a tradesman or farmer, etc. Those

*Persons that cannot be contented with this Liberty that they
have in this Kingdom ... ought to go to the above Countries
abroad and live there and not disturb the Peace and
Happiness of such as are Well-wishers to their King and
Country.*[73]

Just as Katterfelto began this defence of the superiority of the British
Constitution over its revolutionary rival, news of a large meeting of
Dissenters was being reported. It took place under the chairmanship
of William Russell, one of the victims of the riots. Declaring
themselves to be "Enemies to seditious and disorderly practices
under whatever Pretence they are committed", and "Friends to the
Constitution of this Country, on the Principles asserted at the
revolution of 1688, as consisting of King, Lords and Commons",
those present resolved:

*That in Consequence of the abuses which have crept into our
Constitution, they declare themselves warm and zealous
Friends to such a Parliamentary Reform as shall make the
Representation speak the Voice of the People, by rendering
Elections more frequent and the representation more equal.*[74]

Katterfelto responded to this by keeping up the attack for the next
month and declaring himself much surprised at the dissatisfaction of
"a few Persons and Societies" who were calling for parliamentary
reforms. These people seemed to believe that "our Maker and great
King could not guide the King and the Members present of
Parliament to their Benefit". Their political philosophy betrayed a
"Despair as if there were no God in Heaven" and "most of them
must be such that can neither write, or have any Belief in the Bible
or Parliament".[75]

Katterfelto's defence of the realm was populist in tone, which
served the added purpose of trying to draw in the crowds. So he
announced that "as there is a few Persons discontented in this Town,
for Want of better Understanding of the Character of a King, and the
present Members of Parliament" he would deliver once again his
"Lecture on all Characters of Life, from the King to the Beggar".[76]
Those inhabitants of Birmingham who attended the lecture, on the
constitution and liberty of the nation, were later reported to be
astonished, "the Doctor being a Foreigner", to hear him displaying
great talent in the English language.[77]

At the end of January 1793, with the start of the Reign of Terror still some eight months away, Katterfelto was sanguine about the prospects for the royalist cause in France:

> *As Kings, Princes, Dukes, Lords and Parliament-Men are not found in the sea like fishes, nor are they made up in the air like hailstones, Dr KATTERFELTO will therefore lecture every night this week on how the above Noblemen etc. come to their great dignity ... He expects they will have many different Kings at Paris in less than twelve months' time, and as there is a King to guide the whole Universe, the Doctor hopes there will be a Deputy King for many centuries to come in this Country.[78]*

Finally, as Katterfelto prepared to leave Birmingham, which had supported him for such a long time, he expressed his great hope "that this present King George, and his Prussian Majesty will gain the Victory over their Enemies abroad."[79]

His Prussian Majesty made frequent appearances in the British press, not just in news of treaties and wars but also in extracts from his Memoirs. These had been written by Samuel Johnson in 1756 and included such anecdotes as the following item, which appeared three weeks after the storming of the Bastille:

> *The late Frederick was fully sensible of the contagious nature of Liberty. He knew that the spirit of Freedom was epidemical, and he did not chuse to employ his subjects in any way that would put them in the way of catching the disorder. When old Franklin applied to him to lend his assistance to America, "Pray Doctor" says the old veteran, "Pray, Doctor, what is the object they mean to attain?" "Liberty, Sire," replied the Philosopher of Philadelphia, "Liberty! That Freedom which is the birthright of man!" The King, after a short pause, made this memorable and Kingly answer. "I was born a Prince, I am become a King, and I will not use the power which I possess to the ruin of my own trade. I was born to command – and the people were born to obey![80]*

With these anti-revolutionary sentiments Katterfelto would undoubtedly have agreed. Nevertheless, Katterfelto's conservatism was of the compassionate variety. Before he left London in 1784, and being aware of those less fortunate than himself or his audiences, he had demonstrated his Christian charity:

> *Mr KATTERFELTO acquaints all serious and religious persons, that as To-morrow is Good Friday he will make his LECTURES suitable for that day: his Lecture will be on the POWER of the FOUR ELEMENTS, and will shew the Power of Thunder, Lightning, Earthquakes, Winds, and Fire ... The money that will be received is to be distributed to as many distressed persons as have made application to him for it.* [81]

These Good Friday appeals became a regular feature and testified that the moral and divine philosopher practised what he preached. The following year's message focussed on the thousands of Londoners who were in great distress because of "this unhappy war" (i.e. the American War of Independence, which was fast losing any popularity and had just brought the resignation of Lord North's government). In these trying times Katterfelto trusted that all people of good will would join him in helping the unfortunates, remembering our Maker's words: "Those who relieve the poor shall be rewarded, and live in glory in the Kingdom of Heaven for ever and ever."[82]

It was not only the economic sacrifices of wartime that made calls on the charity of the devout Christian. The very cold winters of the mid-1780s, caused in large part by Iceland's volcanic eruptions, created very real problems for the underprivileged. Mindful of this, in the winter of 1784, Katterfelto offered to perform for two nights in aid of the poor, and hoped that

> *several thousand persons in London will have the same humanity and help the distressed; several poor inhabitants have been relieved by him during the extreme cold weather, as he has given in the course of last month upwards of one hundred guineas to the poor; and he flatters himself that these two nights charitable exhibitions will be the means of relieving some hundreds more.* [83]

Such apparent acts of charity were a common feature among travelling showmen. However, all was not always as it seemed. On one occasion his rival Breslaw had promised to use the receipts from a performance to help the poor of Canterbury. He later told the mayor that he had, in fact, divided the money among his company on the grounds that it consisted of those "than whom none could be poorer."[84] In the light of this, Katterfelto's Good Friday appeal for 1784 has a suspicious ring to it:

> *As above 800,000 persons in London have been this week in a great uproar, on account of the contested Election, this being Good Friday, all the money taken will be given to a very distressed family.*[85]

The following year in Norwich, during the run up to Christmas and following his practice "for 24 years past", Katterfelto performed for charity over six nights and announced that after "his day's expenses" the remainder would be given each morning to all those that were in distress. Drawing on the words of the philosopher of Ecclesiastes that "all the world is only Vanity, Vanity and Vanity", he desired that

> *particularly religious persons, and all those who are blessed with health and fortune, will come and see the wonderful works of our Maker and various mechanical powers, and by so doing and helping the distressed, he is in hopes that he and they will be rewarded for it in the Kingdom of Heaven.*[86]

During the 1790s there was a run of poor harvests which resulted in severe food shortages and rocketing prices. In turn, this placed even greater pressure on the system of poor relief provided by parishes. The worst years were 1795 and 96, when riots broke out in many places as people attempted to force millers and bakers to reduce their prices, or else to stop food from leaving the area. The shortage of bread even led soldiers to riot (which caused great concern given the threat of an impending French invasion). Katterfelto rose to the challenge once again. He informed the residents of Gloucester that he was "glad to hear that a resolution is taken to raise a Subscription for the Poor and Distressed families", and declared himself happy to promote "that noble and Christian plan."[87]

Perhaps his Christian piety and generosity were sincere; he certainly hoped that they would be good for business. Either way, the professed object of his lectures remained the intellectual and spiritual enlightenment of his audiences: to impart "a ray which points into the realms divine".[88]

142

What is in Heaven above he does well know,
And if you wish to go there you must hear Katterfelto,
In earth beneath, perhaps in hell too
All is display'd by Monsieur Katterfelto.[89]

Whether it was revealing and explaining the providential wonders of creation, or defending the god-given right of kings to rule, or being an exemplar of Christian charity, the divine and moral philosopher Katterfelto was, "as far as mortal can, ever assisting Heav'ns eternal plan".[90] Indeed, his philosophy was so divine that the greatest comparison of all could be made when his audience "approached him as if they were ambitious to touch even the hem of his garment".[91] His lecture room had become a sacred place, and into it he was willing to "charitably admit all who may have Faith in the Heart and Two Shillings and Six Pence in the Pocket!"[92] It was nothing less than a temple - a temple of learning - and all were bidden to come.

[1] G.J. Whyte-Melville, Katerfelto, 1875, page 55
[2] 5th January 1788, The Caledonian Mercury
[3] 5th January 1788, The Caledonian Mercury
[4] 13th February 1792, Aris's Birmingham Gazette
[5] 16th September 1796, The Iris or Sheffield Advertiser
[6] Thompson Cooper, A New Biographical Dictionary, London, 1873
[7] 6th June 1783, The General Advertiser, op cit; also 17th March 1790, The Cumberland Pacquet
[8] e.g. 2nd July 1792, Aris's Birmingham Gazette
[9] 5th August 1796, The Iris or Sheffield Advertiser
[10] The Mirror of Literature, Amusement and Instruction, op cit
[11] Travels in England in 1782, op cit, page 70
[12] 2nd September 1796, The Iris or Sheffield Advertiser
[13] 5th May 1790, The Cumberland Pacquet
[14] 10th June 1784, The General Advertiser, op cit
[15] 11th March 1793, Aris's Birmingham Gazette
[16] 20th August 1782, The Morning Post
[17] 3rd February 1783, The General Advertiser, op cit
[18] 24th February 1783, The General Advertiser, op cit
[19] 5th April 1784, The General Advertiser, op cit
[20] 6th June 1783, The General Advertiser, op cit
[21] See Chapter 1, page 15
[22] Hird's Annals of Bedale, op cit, page 222
[23] 14th July 1787, The Newcastle Courant
[24] 21st July 1787, The Newcastle Courant

[25] The Rambler Magazine, 145, August 6th 1751

[26] 30th January 1792, Aris's Birmingham Gazette; also 16th December 1786, The Leeds Mercury and 9th December 1789, The Cumberland Pacquet

[27] 19th July 1782, The Morning Post

[28] 2nd December 1782, The Morning Post

[29] 29th December 1783, The General Advertiser, op cit

[30] 26th April 1784, The General Advertiser, op cit

[31] 25th April 1791, Williamson's Liverpool Advertiser

[32] 14th November 1791, Williamson's Liverpool Advertiser; 6th August 1794, The Hereford Journal

[33] 29th December 1783, The General Advertiser, op cit

[34] See Dava Sobel's "Longitude", Fourth Estate, London, 1996, pages 41-43

[35] 29th December 1783, The General Advertiser, op cit

[36] 12th December 1786, The York Courant, 17th March 1790, The Cumberland Pacquet

[37] 6th August 1783, The General Advertiser, op cit, also 14th November 1782, The General Advertiser, op cit

[38] 3rd November 1783, The General Advertiser, op cit

[39] 10th November 1783, The Morning Post

[40] 20th August 1783, The General Advertiser, op cit

[41] 15th July 1796, The Iris or Sheffield Advertiser

[42] 23rd-26th October 1781, The Edinburgh Advertiser

[43] 1st December 1794, The Gloucester Journal; 2nd April 1796, The Nottingham Journal

[44] 20th August 1783, The General Advertiser, op cit

[45] 5th April 1782, The Morning Post

[46] 20th August 1783, The General Advertiser, op cit

[47] 25th February 1784, The Morning Post; and 31st January 1788, The Caledonian Mercury

[48] 14th November 1782, The General Advertiser, op cit

[49] 6th August 1783, The General Advertiser, op cit

[50] 29th December 1783, The General Advertiser, op cit

[51] 19th June 1784, The General Advertiser, op cit

[52] 26th April 1784, The General Advertiser, op cit

[53] Erke Energy Research and Engineering Corporation, www.en.wikipedia.org/wiki/History_of_perpetual_motion_machines

[54] Quoted in Thomas Frost, op cit, chapter 6

[55] 10th June 1784, The General Advertiser, op cit

[56] 5th May, 24th May, 5th June 1784, The General Advertiser, op cit

[57] 24th June 1784, The General Advertiser, op cit

[58] 27th January 1790, The Cumberland Pacquet

[59] 18th October 1793, The Shrewsbury Chronicle

[60] 22nd October 1795, The Derby Mercury

[61] 27th February 1796, The Nottingham Journal

[62] 5th August 1796, The Iris or Sheffield Advertiser

[63] 16th January 1797, The York Courant

[64] 27th February 1796, The Nottingham Journal

[65] 11th January 1792, The Wolverhampton Chronicle

[66] "Essay on Quackery", op cit

[67] RB Rose, The Priestly Riots of 1791, Past and Present, 18 (1960) pages 68-88

[68] 27th February 1792, Aris's Birmingham Gazette

[69] 10th February 1790, The Cumberland Pacquet

[70] 14th April 1781, The Morning Post

[71] 16th April 1781, The Morning Chronicle

[72] 28th May and 10th December 1792, Aris's Birmingham Gazette

[73] 24th December 1792, Aris's Birmingham Gazette

[74] 24th December 1792, Aris's Birmingham Gazette

[75] 31st December 1792, Aris's Birmingham Gazette

[76] 7th January 1793, Aris's Birmingham Gazette

[77] 21st January 1793, Aris's Birmingham Gazette

[78] 28th January 1793, Aris's Birmingham Gazette

[79] 1st April 1793, Aris's Birmingham Gazette

[80] 7th-10th August 1789, The Glasgow Mercury

[81] 12th April 1781, The Morning Post

[82] 29th March 1782, The Morning Herald

[83] 7th February 1784, The Morning Post

[84] Quoted in Thomas Frost, op cit, chapter 7

[85] 9th April 1784, The General Advertiser, op cit

[86] 18th December 1785, The Norfolk Chronicle

[87] 12th January 1794, The Gloucester Journal

[88] 6th September 1782, The Morning Post

[89] 5th August 1782, The Morning Post

[90] 23rd-26th October 1787, The Edinburgh Advertiser

[91] 8th August 1782, The Morning Post

[92] 25th August 1798, The Newcastle Courant

CHAPTER 7

THE FASHIONABLE TEMPLE OF INSTRUCTION

We understand that His Royal Highness Prince Florestan,who has been for some little time in this country, has taken the mansion in Carlton Gardens, recently occupied by the Marquis of Katterfelto. Benjamin Disraeli, "Endymion", chapter 45, 1880

Katterfelto had many peers: travelling entertainers, travelling lecturers, travelling medical irregulars and travelling balloonists. Few, if any of them, could match the combination of "wonders" that he presented. None came anywhere near him for the quantity, persistence, and sheer audacity of his publicity.

As a master of the art of puffing Katterfelto always aimed for both height and breadth. He strove to be associated with the nobility: what he called the "ladies and gentlemen of the first rank". Yet he also knew that he needed to attract people from every walk of life: those in the professions, the labourers and the servants. He needed them all if he was to continue to make a living and keep his name on people's lips. However, he faced a great deal of competition attracting an audience. In addition to his many rivals he had to contend with a whole host of other entertainments, for over the paper at breakfast people could discuss whether to go to the theatre, take in a blood sport or visit a freak show.

The social capital of Britain was London and everyone who could afford it went up to the city at least once a year. Londoners themselves were very proud of their new parks and it was in these that the social round began each day. In particular it was to Hyde Park that the well-to-do flocked for "the Fashionable Hour". This public promenade was actually three hours long, beginning at 4.30pm although ladies didn't usually appear until later. Then it was home in time for dinner at 7.30pm, or earlier if a trip to the theatre (or Katterfelto's show) was planned. Evenings at the theatre were long affairs - curtain up was at 6.30pm - and they often ended around midnight, or even later. As one German lady visiting London in 1786 observed: "Up to eleven o'clock at night there are as many people along the street as at Frankfurt during the fair, not to mention the eternal stream of coaches."[1]

Some of these coaches were privately owned (like the one, newly made at a cost of some £3000, which Katterfelto boasted would be the grandest in London).[2] Others were the Hackney Coaches, who took their name from the French "haquenee" meaning "horse for hire". By the 1770s there were about a thousand of these one-horse chaises ferrying people around the streets of London: sufficient numbers in fact for them already to be licensed and have a number plate. On dark nights a far cheaper but much more risky journey home was with the aid of a "link boy". A farthing paid for a boy who carried a flaming pitch torch (with a burning cotton wick, or "link"). However, some of these boys turned out to be "moon-cursers", leading people into the hands of robbers. Their name came from the fact that when there was sufficient moonlight there was no need for people to take the risk and hire one of them, hence they cursed the moon.

By now London's theatres were vast, holding two to three thousand people and almost every provincial town had its own playhouse. Some of the stately homes also had their own domestic theatres. Troupes of players toured the country and some actors made great names for themselves, such as David Garrick and Mrs. Siddons. Gone were the days of satirical and racy Restoration plays. In came gentle, sentimental and moralising comedies appealing to the less intellectual middle-classes. Many were musical farces or pantomimes, like those which had parodied both Dr. Graham and Katterfelto.

Instead of the theatre, anyone searching for something new could visit Astley's "Amphitheatre Riding School" near Westminster Bridge. Philip Astley, "the English Hussar" of the gun trick fame, was an ex-cavalry man who, as well as conjuring, performed many daredevil riding stunts and adopted the circular ring as a way to enable his audiences to view them (rather than him riding off into the distance). To his feats of horsemanship Astley added other elements, common to fairgrounds of the day, which were to become synonymous with later ideas of the circus. There were "pantomimical, farcical, tragical, and operatical performances" by clowns on horseback. There was tumbling, rope vaulting and ladder jumping. There were "the beautiful Zebra", "the Camel or Dromedary from Grand Cairo, and the Elk from Bombay".[3] And there were the horses themselves, who performed tricks such as sitting up and lying down to the sound of a trumpet and dancing a Minuet or Hornpipe.[4] Astley also added pantomimes and musical numbers to create a show of great variety that changed with the seasons.

He was soon being imitated in London by the "Royal Circus and Equestrian Academy" and it was this establishment, rather than Astley's Amphitheatre, that bequeathed the name of "circus" to this form of entertainment. (Katterfelto took a swipe at these spectacles when he announced that his Black Cat would entertain people "in a manner far superior to any Theatrical, Equestrian, or Tumbling Exhibition whatsoever.")[5]

If people didn't roll up to the circus then they could visit one of the many "curiosities" that abounded at that time. There was, for instance, Mr. Nicholson and his "Learned Pig", which appeared at the Saddler's Wells Theatre in 1784 and went on to tour the provinces. Audiences could witness Nicholson's "exclusive and peculiar power over the most irrational part of animated nature... his persevering temper and patience in the tuition of Beasts, Birds etc". The proof of this ability lay in his having taught

a Turtle to fetch and carry; his overcoming the timidity of a HARE by making her beat a drum; his perfecting six TURKEY COCKS in a regular country-dance; his completing a small BIRD in the performance of many surprising feats; his having taught three CATS to strike several times on the dulcimer with their paw and to imitate the Italians in the manner of their singing; but above all, his conquering the natural obstinacy and stupidity of a PIG, by teaching him to write the letters of any person's name, the number of persons in the room, the hour and minute by any watch, etc. etc.[6]

Other curiosities were exhibited of a more truly educational nature. People could indulge their general fascination with all things electrical by viewing "the Electrical Eel from Surinam", which was on tour in the late 1770s. Of particular interest to the scientifically minded was that this creature could give out shocks and flashes of light exactly like the static electricity held in a Leyden jar. The publicity for this exhibition claimed that the eel had been exhibited to seventy gentlemen who all received a shock at the same time.[7]

There were many human curiosities as well. Count Borulasaki, a Polish dwarf, had come to Britain in the 1780s at the invitation of the British Ambassador to Vienna. He performed in London and throughout Scotland and Ireland, giving concerts on the violin and playing his own compositions. Borulasaki became so successful that the King of Poland withdrew the allowance on which he had previously been living. At the other extreme was Patrick Cotter, otherwise known as "the Irish Giant", who claimed to be nine feet tall and hoped "with the blessing of God, to grow some feet higher."[8] Alternatively, in 1787 Londoners could be shocked and amazed by "three Wild-born human beings each with a Monstrous Craw ... under their throats". Said to be the offspring of Hannibal's elephants, they were in fact three visiting South Americans who suffered from very enlarged goitres.[9]

In this culture of curiosity, people could even stay at home and indulge their fascination for all things "MIRACULOUS! QUEER! ODD! STRANGE! SUPERNATURAL! WHIMSICAL! ABSURD! OUT OF THE WAY! AND UNACCOUNTABLE!" by reading "The New Wonderful Magazine". With endless tales of all that was "STRANGE and yet most TRUE" it was dedicated to bringing its readers news of "the most surprising escapes from death; Deliverance from Dangers; Strange Discoveries of long-concealed Murders; Dreadful Shipwrecks; accounts of persons famous for Eating, Drinking, Fasting, Walking or Sleeping...and whatever else is calculated to promote Mirth or Astonishment or that is Wonderful and Miraculous." In short the magazine was designed "to charm a WONDERING AGE".[10]

If one tired of curiosities, though frankly people never seemed to, a widespread form of entertainment was available to those who went down to their local inn, or to the many coffee-houses or occasional "chocolate-house" to play what Katterfelto called "destructive billiards".[11] This was emerging into something like the modern game and it could be played for large sums of money. Gambling of all kinds was a national obsession, with wagers being laid on just about anything imaginable: from cards to horses, from drinking pints of gin to eating live cats, from the death of the king to the national lottery (which ran from 1709 to 1824).[12]

Then there was always a bit of sport to set the blood racing. Organised fox-hunting made its debut in Georgian Britain and newspapers regularly advertised "A Main of Cocks". Cockfighting was very widespread. Every sizeable town had its own cockpit; the one in Hyde Park could even call itself "the Cockpit Royal". People of all social classes would attend and would bet large sums of money on the outcome, which was usually the death of one of the birds, killed by the spurs of metal or bone which were strapped to the birds' feet. Another very violent sport was boxing. In an age before the Marquis of Queensbury, this was just anything goes, last man standing, street fighting, and was often watched by crowds of thousands. The fighting wasn't always confined to the contestants either, with "audience participation" breaking out during or after the fight.

It was an unruly age when violence was commonplace. Entertainers (and audiences) needed to take account of this, as one visitor to the Haymarket Theatre recalled: "Every moment a rotten orange came whizzing past me or past my neighbour; one hit my hat, but I dared not turn round for fear one hit me in the face."[13] Katterfelto's audiences certainly got out of hand at times, and in response he devised his own form of defence:

Here the drunken bucks, or frothy fools, unwilling to improve, and unable to amend, kick up a dust, to prevent those who are desirous of both, and madly break or meanly pilfer some of the apparatus they are not capable of discerning the use of; till the Philosopher, forgetting the first principle of his profession, a command of temper, breaks out into a paroxysm of rage, vented half in English, half in German, puts on the terrific Death's Head Hussars cap and the rusty sword wore by his grandfather the General, when he took 30,000 prisoners, till the champion of confusion, ashamed of meanness, or afraid of punishment, hastily decamping, he re-assumes his lecture.[14]

Sometimes the aggressive or disgruntled customers followed Katterfelto home. On one occasion when this happened he announced that he hoped

no person will come to Dr Katterfelto's house at night as well as by day, as a certain Clerk to a Banker at Charing Cross did, with his companions, on Thursday night...otherwise such persons can expect the course of law.[15]

Fortunately there were exceptions to this rowdy conduct and Katterfelto took every opportunity to let it be known when he

150

thought that an audience had behaved well. In 1792, "Above 150 of Lord Dudley's Gentlemen, Tradesmen, Clerks and Miners" had been to see some of Katterfelto's "Philosophical Experiments" in Dudley Town Hall. The whole company had behaved with "greatest Politeness", which was something that gave the Doctor more pleasure "than all the Money he has received by his various Lectures during the fourteen days he has been at Dudley".[16] Likewise in Birmingham he expressed thanks to a large party "for their Company and Encouragement, but more so for their genteel Behaviour, as they did behave to him as complete Ladies and Gentlemen."[17]

Katterfelto certainly worked hard to attract people from polite society. As coaches were the way to travel for the well off, Katterfelto regularly made it clear which class of people he was hoping to see by encouraging coaches to arrive early:

> *Mr Katterfelto humbly begs the favour of the Nobility and Gentry who are pleased to favour him with their company, to give orders to their coachmen to draw back from the bottom of Spring Gardens so as to allow other carriages to come up to the door.*[18]

He also regularly expressed regret that large numbers of ladies and gentlemen had arrived too late to gain admittance. To avoid disappointment he advised people that "it will therefore be necessary for Ladies and Gentlemen to send their servants at five o'clock to keep places, and to send for their tickets one or two days before."[19]

In attracting the right sort of clientele Katterfelto found it helpful to let others know that "a Gentleman had dropped a White Purse, with Three Guineas in gold and a Note of Hand for £2000 payable to Capt. Baterson".[20] The Captain was later able to express his gratitude for Katterfelto's "genteel behaviour" in returning his property, "which shows great honour and honesty", even more so as Katterfelto had declined a reward for his action.[21] Katterfelto did though let it slip that "Captain Petterson" (another casualty of the accent) after having recovered the money "was very polite to leave £1 7s, but the different adverts cost Katterfelto £2 5s."[22]

Although 1783 saw him adopting the persona of "Colonel Katterfelto", this was merely a brief flirtation; he dropped the title the following year. Colonel or not, he found himself entertaining the troops for many years to come. He reported that Admiral Sir Peter

Parker, the head of the navy, and General Conway, the army commander in chief, had both attended his shows,[23] as had His Royal Highness Prince William of Gloucester and the officers of his regiment at Gloucester.[24] The officers from various regiments billeted around the country, such as Colonel and Lady Stroud together with "the greatest part of the Gentlemen Officers of the Somersetshire Cavalry" were all reported to have spent profitable and enjoyable evenings in Katterfelto's company.[25]

As well as the military, there were the politicians: Pitt the Younger,[26] Lord North (just after he had resigned as Prime Minister)[27] and various other Lords in high office as well as, in later years, the mayors of York, Oswestry and Nottingham. The nobility invited Katterfelto into their stately homes: he entertained Her Royal Highness the Princess de Crenne (or Cronne) at Arley Hall, and Lady Winn and her guests for five nights at Nostell Priory.[28] The children of the gentry were also invited into his temple of learning: "Young ladies or gentlemen at Boarding Schools, if 20 or 30 in Number, will be admitted at 1s."[29]

Nor should we think that all these claims were mere puffery. The social life of the nation often involved the mixing of all levels of society and all were drawn into the ubiquitous culture of curiosity. For example, in 1783 the European Magazine reported that both the Archbishop of Canterbury and Dr. Johnson had paid visits to Katterfelto (although it indicated that their response was one of "risibility in all degrees").[30] With this sort of popularity, or at least with this level of interest to see what all the fuss was about, it is no wonder that Katterfelto was soon able to express his great pleasure on hearing that, within polite circles, his exhibition room had acquired the title of "the Morning Promenade and the Fashionable Temple of Instruction".[31]

From the summer of 1782 Katterfelto was even more delighted to announce that since his arrival in London he had been honoured with the presence of royalty. In the October he took pleasure in announcing that "If the weather prove fine next week, the King, Queen, Prince of Wales and all the Royal Family intend to see those great Wonders which are now exhibiting with his Solar Microscope".[32] Although poor weather delayed this event until November, Katterfelto hoped that the King and Prince of Wales would be coming to see him once again within a few days.[33]

Throughout 1783 he regularly let it be known that the whole Royal Family had witnessed his wonders and had expressed their "highest satisfaction",[34] with the Doctor having been "much taken notice of".[35] Katterfelto delighted in being a particular favourite of the Prince of Wales, later to be George IV, although on his second visit in the spring the prince had been disappointed (unbelievably) "for want of room".[36] So, by the beginning of 1784 the entertainer was able to boast that he was a great friend of his Majesty the King and the whole Royal Family, and later puffed that he had performed for them as many as eight times.[37]

These sorts of claims were common among Katterfelto's fellow "philosopher-magicians". Pinetti had "a written testimony of his Majesty's approbation, signed with his own hand and certificates of the same nature from several other Sovereigns".[38] Breslaw claimed to have performed several times for their Majesties as well as appearing three times by royal command of the Prince of Wales during the summer of 1787 in "Brighthelmstone";[39] (a little fishing port, made popular by the Prince for sea bathing, which later became far better known as Brighton). Despite large quantities of hot air, all this is actually not so unlikely or outlandish as it sounds. Through this period the Royal Family flirted with populism, regularly visiting fairs until the late 1780s, and getting caught up in "balloonmania" like everyone else. Along with their counterparts on the Continent they may well have invited the entertainers of the moment to exhibit before them.

Katterfelto, though, was not content simply to be the favourite of British royalty but announced that his fame was drawing the attention of other royal houses. The first signs of this were the appearances in 1783 of several "foreign ministers" and "emissaries from the several potentates of Europe, who are sent by their respective Courts to attend his lectures".[40] One such courtier was the Duke de Chartres,[41] a French libertine whose great fondness for all things British brought the disapproval of his kinsman Louis XVI.[42](The Duke's revenge in later years was to vote for the guillotining of the King.) As a result of the reports submitted by these noble reviewers, the interest of the royal courts was declared to have grown to fever pitch. In February, the London papers carried an "Extract from a letter from the Paris Gazette" which declared,

There never was in this city a greater desire for the presence of any man, than for the celebrated Katterfelto. Comte de Grasse has spoken so much of his merit that the King and Queen are very anxious to see Mr. Katterfelto's exhibition.[43]

The Queen was reported to have a gold snuffbox inlaid with diamonds waiting for the great philosopher when he arrived,[44]while the King of France had sent him "a very handsome present", expressing a wish that Katterfelto would visit Paris on his way to Berlin.[45] The reason for the trip to Berlin was that the King of Prussia had supposedly chosen this most illustrious of philosophers, above all his peers, to exhibit some of his wonders before His Majesty.[46] In June an extract from a letter from Berlin announced that

> The King of Prussia has taken very great notice of his Royal Highness the Prince Bishop of Osnaburg since his arrival at Potsdam ... And the King of Prussia is very proud to hear that [Katterfelto] is the most complete man for a field of battle.[47]

This military prowess might come in handy as by now the growing rivalry between the Courts of Berlin and Paris for the favours of the great man threatened to endanger the fragile peace in Europe:

> We are informed that Katterfelto is not only the greatest philosopher that ever lived, but that a most bloody war is likely to take place between the Kings of France and Prussia, contending for the honour of having the said philosopher at Versailles or Berlin; to the latter he is bound, by duty, to return speedily, but, at the special request of his Most Christian Majesty, and the earnest solicitations of Doctor Franklin, he intends to visit the latter, should not the British Court interfere, for his continuance in this Metropolis, which we may believe is the very business that retards forming a new Administration.[48]

As it turned out, Katterfelto decided to remain in London, so Europe was spared a new war and Britain was saved from anarchy, with the formation of the Fox-North coalition. (The real reason for the delay in creating a new administration was that George III vehemently hated Fox and viewed North as a traitor, and so he was busy trying, unsuccessfully, to persuade Pitt the Younger to become prime minister.)

As for the Kings of Europe, they took the attitude that if the mountain will not come to Mohammed them Mohammed must go to the mountain. In October 1783 mysterious French noblemen started appearing at Katterfelto's shows:

They have attended his Lectures eighteen succeeding nights, also several times in the daytime. ... One of these Noblemen, it is said, is a very great personage ... Dr Katterfelto received great salary last Saturday, a very handsome Order of St Louis, set with diamonds, from the Great Personage; he also promised the Doctor a settlement if he would come to Paris. If that great personage is the King of France, as was confidently reported by several French Gentlemen, Dr Katterfelto says he is not the first King in the World who travelled in disguise; as the present King of Prussia also the King of Poland does so very often, which is more to their honour than disgrace, as Dr Katterfelto says, as a Divine and Moral Philosopher, that wisdom increases in a person by hearing, seeing, travelling and studying.[49]

Clearly, Katterfelto was having a great deal of fun with this strand of puffery. Although he let royal "Katterfelto-mania" die down it did not go away altogether. Indeed he allowed it to spread slowly but surely eastward until, by the early 1790s, it had reached the Ottoman Empire, as the good folk of Chester were to learn when their local rag carried a most surprising letter from the Sultan himself:

Copy of a letter from the grand Signior to the most renowned, sublime and wonderful Doctor Katterfelto. Achmet, Magnus and Optimus.
Illustrious Man!
As mortals desire the light on the sun, so do mine eyes thirst after thee! Thy presence will be refreshing unto me, as the soft zephyrs in the Garden of Eden. Enter, then, the land of my dominions, and let thy feet touch the threshold of my palace; for thou shalt be received as a Vizir, and treated as one of the princes. The nobles of Turkey shall bow the knee unto thee, and even the doors of my Seraglio shall open at the breach of thy lips. Hear, and be compassionate, oh! illustrious man, the sorrows that have preyed on the commander of the faithful, on the almighty Lord of Europe. As the pomegranate tree withereth when the casements of heaven are closed, and as the soft flower descending in the evening refresheth the same, so did the Sovereign of Constantinople languish for the presence of the incomparable Katterfelto, and so will thy

arrival revive my spirit within me. To turn the current of affliction, I have built an ebony palace for my beloved Sultana Zoraide, and have called it the wonderful Wonder of Wonders. That lovely flower of the creation having brought me a son, fair as the early dawn that gilds the mountains of the east, I have caused him to be named Katterfelto. This is what I ask of thee in return, let not thy ear hear with complacency – let not thine heart deny my request: when the black cat that is the partner of thy wisdom, and of thy fame, and falsely is called The Prince of Darkness; when thy cat shall bless thy ravished soul with a progeny black as the sable eyes of Mahomet, Oh! let her first born be named Achmet. Haste thee, oh! illustrious man, and come and embrace me. By thy mighty assistance shall I discomfit all my foes, yet shalt thou not draw thy scymitar to slay them. Thou shalt be at the head of my Janiferies [elite troops made up of Christian eunuchs], and all the warriors of mine host shall follow thee. At my right hand shall stand thy black cat and the young kitten Achmet; before thee shall be placed thy great solar microscope, which representing thee and thine army to mine enemies of an horrible magnitude, the terror of thine appearance will send them to the shades below. Let love of glory inflame thy breast, and make thee quit the land in which thou sojournest, or by the great toe of Mahomet I will send the Aga of the Janiferies, and the Baska of the Sea, to cut off the tail of thy cat, and to burn all the occult secrets that thou shalt have committed to paper. But if thou obeyest my commands, the taper of affection shall ever burn for thee in the breast of ACHMET

As if this was not enough to melt the heart of the most reluctant philosopher, the letter was followed by a short poetic offering:

Hail learned sage, whose philosophical lore
Can point out wonders never known before!
Hail, magic cat, whose more than mortal rump
Now boasts a tail, and now has not a stump!
Come, sage and cat, your rapid footsteps bend
To Turkey's Lord, your patron and your friend,
The sage, the Sultan, and the sable cat,
Shall form the third and best triumvirate;

Admiring eyes shall adore thy name,
And the grand trio gain immortal fame![50]

Surely this was one of the high points of Katterfelto's puffing, but he was keen to show that what mattered was not just the quality of his fans but their quantity as well. By the summer of 1783 he was claiming that more than 96,100 Londoners (or one tenth of the city's population) had been to see his exhibition.[51] On his travels he was supposedly often performing to "many crowded houses with great applause",[52] while in Grantham his popularity was such as to create logistical problems for the town:

> *The oldest Man living in this Town cannot remember that any Person in a public way of life ever surprised our Nobility so much before as the above wonderful Philosopher ... Many country Ladies and Gentlemen of sixty and seventy Years of age have come to Grantham on his account, which have not been to this Town for many Years before, and it is expected if the Doctor stays here much longer that no Beds will be had at any Inn for Money.*[53]

Judging the true size of Katterfelto's audiences is difficult. The people of Birmingham do seem to have received him particularly favourably, given that he remained there profitably for a year: far and away the longest period he performed anywhere outside of London. However, even the man himself acknowledged that at first his welcome in the town had not been universal:

> *As for some of those Gentlemen we find, that were the Doctor's greatest Enemies on his first Arrival in this Town, become now his best Friends.*[54]

He was soon claiming that there was "hardly one Hour of the Day but some of the above Gentlemen are with him; the Doctor is also much in favour with the Ladies."[55]

Such was his apparent celebrity status in Birmingham that towards the end of his stay he introduced into his merchandising a very personal memento of his shows. The audience could take away with them "his likeness in the same Character as he delivers his Evening Lectures, they may have them now ... at the low Price of One Shilling ... as natural as Life."[56] (This "likeness" sounds very much like a copy of the picture that had appeared in the European Magazine some ten years before. See illustration 2.) York may have been another place that received him well. He clocked up three visits there over the years, which lends some support to his claim that "he is a great favourite there, particularly among the Ladies".[57]

Elsewhere, though, Katterfelto bemoaned the lack of response that he encountered in certain communities and praised the "Thrice happy few, who wisely here attend".[58] Fairly typical was his accusation, laid at the door of the people of Nottingham, that "the greater part of the inhabitants of this opulent and populace place will have to repent they let slip the opportunity of beholding the effects of his incomparable Solar Microscope".[59] His visit to Stafford in 1991 appears to have been the all-time low point. Over eight nights, not a single person attended his show.[60] The poor weather and the constant flow of ridicule over the years, including several swipes by the popular satirical poet Peter Pindar,[61] undoubtedly took its toll around the country. However, another motivation for many people staying away was that they had a religious objection to his shows:

> *Dr Katterfelto is much surprised and astonished that those persons who dress very plain, and profess to be very religious and are able to see, and are not blind, and can well afford, do not enjoy our Maker's great handy-works, so much as those who are called gay and dressy people who have the good sense and grace…and do not look on a philosopher to be a false prophet and teacher, as the Jews did our Saviour in Jerusalem, and not make their money their god.*[62]

The "very religious" were reacting against Katterfelto's "natural philosophy", preferring instead the biblical revelation at the heart of the religious revival which was sweeping the country. There was a theological and ethical gulf between Katterfelto's High Church Tory views and the Low Church radicalism of many Evangelicals. In Chester this led one Evangelical to take up Katterfelto's catchphrase – not to praise him but to lambast, as gullible and hedonistic, those who turned up to this sort of show:

> *Wonders!!! – not produced by the magnifying aid of the Solar Microscope.*

It is wonderful to see men of great landed and personal property, of ancient family and established integrity, nose-led by dicers, carders, adventurers and swindlers!

It is wonderful to see characters denominated gentlemen spending their time in pursuit of pleasures which can neither produce them honour or enjoyment!

The writer then turned his attack to the morality of the day, giving us a glimpse of the ethical stance of this new religious movement:

It is wonderful that women whom Heaven hath endowed with grace and beauty, should effect deformity in dress, false colourings in complexion, and make themselves disgusting from an intention to appear amiable!

It is wonderful that men, forgetting the dignity of their station on earth, should degenerate into effeminacy, and assume to manners of the doubtful gender!

It is wonderful to see effeminacy in breeches and masculine affection under petticoats!

Having had a good go at the familiar territory of gender and sexuality, he then turned his attention to social problems, showing something of the reforming agenda that was strongly associated with the emerging Evangelical movement:

It is wonderful to see men of rank and fortune personally countenance the savage practice of boxing – the stages of which are crowded, whilst our churches are empty!

It is wonderful to see men, which profess humanity and Christian forbearance, implacably keep their unfortunate fellow-creatures for a long series of years in prison – as the best mode of compelling them to pay their debts!

It is wonderful to see men of common sense spending their money, and what is more valuable, their time, in taverns and ale-houses, which would be much better employed in cultivating their own families interests!

After this public tirade it is not surprising that the author preferred to remain anonymous. Having concluded his sarcastic litany of "wonders" he added a final twist by signing himself: "Katterfelto".[63]

The true Katterfelto was probably never going to win around the strict Evangelicals. With others he used reason, and an appeal to his usefulness, to try to persuade the mind. When this failed, he turned to poetry to move the heart and open the pocket. One such poem was published towards the end of his life, during a visit to Sheffield. It has a rather sad and pensive feel, yet its criticism of those who were staying away was hardly likely to endear him to his readers. Even so, it neatly sums up so much about his target audience over the decades:

Ye wise men of Sheffield, and all ye religious,
How long shall the Doctor thus court you in vain?
Come, come to his lectures, and don't be litigious,
But cheerfully join in his wonderful train;
Ye folks of all sizes with cash in your pockets
Why stand ye thus gazing, ye know not at what?
Come, see great Katterfelto,
The Prince of Philosophers, and his Black Cat.

Ye Masons! possessing such secrets and wonders,
A lesson to you, let the Doctor impart;
He'll soon disentangle your system of blunders,
And clearly unravel the brotherly art;
But why then so slow in attending the Doctor,
When lo! a whole fortnight for you he has sat?
Come, see great Katterfelto,
The Prince of Philosophers, and his Black Cat.

Be astonish'd, ye Doctors who deal in prescriptions,
Attend to instruction, that you may be wise,
With old and young surgeons, of ev'ry description,
For this is the man what will open your eyes;
He'll make all the crammers of drugs so asham'd,
That they'll fall on their faces before him, quite flat.
Come, see great Katterfelto,
The Prince of Philosophers, and his Black Cat.

Ye Churchmen! especially ye learned Clergy,
He calls to be teachable and bend at his knee,
He'll from all gross Ideas in divinity purge ye,
And with his bright eye-salve, soon make you to see;

Let none therefore preach of the world that's above,
Nor ramble, nor rant with their spiritual chat,
Till they've seen the great Katterfelto
The Prince of Philosophers, and his Black Cat.

Ye people demure in plain coat and bonnet
He wonders that you should neglect him so long,
He thinks if you've money, you make a god on it,
And so you must be an idolatrous throng;
But why should you doubt of the Doctor's devotion,
By's gown, or his band, or the cut of his hat,
'Till you've seen the great Katterfelto,
The Prince of Philosophers, and his Black Cat.

Ye ladies! who shine (like the sun so auspicious)
On learning, and talents, wherever they be;
Shine now in full splendour, and don't be capricious,
But draw out your purse, and deliver the fee;
Your approaches to Tabby will then be regarded,
The Doctor will also look pleasant at that;
Then you'll quite ravish the great Katterfelto,
The Prince of Philosophers, and his Black Cat.[64]

[1] Sophie von la Roche, in "Sophie in London", 1786
[2] 6th August 1783, The General Advertiser, op cit
[3] 31st March 1781 and 25th July 1782, The Morning Post
[4] 23rd January 1783, The Daily Advertiser
[5] 28th July 1783, The Morning Post
[6] 2nd-9th May 1787, The Glasgow Mercury
[7] 28th July 1777 Aris's Birmingham Gazette
[8] 18th April 1792, The Wolverhampton Chronicle
[9] 21st September and 20th October 1787, The Morning Herald
[10] 7th February 1794, The Hereford Journal
[11] e.g. 19th March 1796, The Nottingham Journal
[12] Roy Porter, "English Society in the 18th Century", page 238, Penguin, 1991.
[13] Karl Philipp Moritz, op cit, page 61
[14] 6th June 1783, The General Advertiser, op cit
[15] 30th August 1783, The General Advertiser, op cit
[16] 19th March 1792, Aris's Birmingham Gazette
[17] 29th October 1792, Aris's Birmingham Gazette
[18] e.g. 6th March 1782, The Morning Post

19 24th December 1784, The Norfolk Chronicle

20 5th March 1783, The Morning Post

21 11th March 1783, The Morning Post

22 26th March 1783, The Morning Chronicle

23 31st October 1782, The Morning Post

24 2nd February 1794, The Gloucester Journal

25 21st May 1795, Berrow's Worcester Journal; also 19th December 1786, The Leeds Intelligencer and 12th November 1795, The Derby Mercury

26 9th December 1789, The Cumberland Pacquet

27 1st April 1782, The Morning Post

28 See the Appendix

29 14th March 1791, Williamson's Liverpool Advertiser

30 The European Magazine, op cit

31 1st May 1783, The Morning Chronicle

32 4th and 9th October 1782, The Morning Post

33 14th November 1782, The Morning Herald

34 e.g. 29th January, The Morning Chronicle

35 19th July 1783, The General Advertiser, op cit

36 26th March 1783 The Morning Chronicle; April 17th 1783, The General Advertiser, op cit

37 14th-17th August 1787, The Edinburgh Advertiser; 5th August 1788, Aberdeen Journal

38 2nd November 1784, The Morning Post

39 18th August 1788, The Aberdeen Journal

40 6th June 1783, The General Advertiser, op cit

41 e.g. 16th May 1783, The Morning Post

42 27th August 1785 Cambridge Chronicle

43 3rd February 1783, The General Advertiser, op cit

44 28th March 1783, The General Advertiser, op cit

45 17th February 1783, The General Advertiser, op cit

46 14th November 1782, The Morning Herald

47 5th June 1783, The General Advertiser, op cit

48 28th March 1783, The General Advertiser, op cit

49 14th October 1783, The Morning Chronicle

50 14th January 1791, The Chester Chronicle

51 19th July 1783, The Morning Chronicle

52 e.g. 24th December 1784, The Norfolk Chronicle

53 10th February 1786, The Lincoln, Rutland and Stamford Mercury

54 14th May 1792, Aris's Birmingham Gazette

55 23rd April 1792, Aris's Birmingham Gazette

56 5th November 1792, Aris's Birmingham Gazette; see also 18th March 1793

57 12th October 1786, The York Courant

58 30th August 1796, The Sheffield Courant

59 13th February 1796, The Nottingham Journal

[60] 19th March 1792, Aris's Birmingham Gazette
[61] Article on Katterfelto in The Dictionary of National Biography, volume 30, 1892
[62] 14th January 1791, The Chester Chronicle
[63] 14th & 28th January 1791, The Chester Chronicle
[64] 27th September 1796, The Sheffield Courant

CHAPTER 8

THE FINAL CURTAIN

*"Katterfelto wishes that his Name, as well as his Merit,
may be remembered for these hundred Years to come."*
The General Advertiser, 5th May 1784

In the autumn of 1799, Katterfelto took to the stage for the last time.
He had been travelling for the whole of his adult life. He had
performed on most days of the week, twice a day or more, for
twenty-three years, with perhaps another fifteen on the Continent.
That amounts to well over 15,000 shows. Through that time he had
puffed his way onto the pages of most of the newspapers in Britain.
He had assumed many persona: the greatest philosopher, the
cleverest conjuror, the healer of untold ills, the man of mystery and
dark powers, the pious and philanthropic Christian, the valiant
explorer of the skies, the most useful man in the kingdom, and
others. He had frequently been ridiculed and vilified on stage, in
cartoons, in song and in print. He had lost his temper with hecklers,
rivals and challengers. He had weathered the hardships of the road
and felt the force of the law. Occasionally, and worst of all, he had
simply been ignored.

There must have been easier ways to make a living and provide
for his wife and children. But then that has probably always been the
case for travelling showmen and women. No doubt, like them, what
kept him going was partly that he knew no other way of life, but
above all it was the thrill of the performance. Because, for all the
ridicule, some of it certainly justified, he had also entertained and
instructed countless thousands of people, introducing them to
"Wonders! Wonders! and Wonders!" Sometimes they didn't just
laugh mockingly at him but genuinely enjoyed the show, gazed in
awe, and learnt much from it. Among these were the people of
Bedale with whom he spent his last days.

By the time he arrived at his final resting place the black "apprentices" were long gone. They may well have been trying to go for some time. At Kendal in 1790 Katterfelto let it be known that one of them (and one of his cats) had left his employ:

> *But the Doctor is likely to be instrumental of propagating more knowledge in foreign parts than all the millions that have been furnished by the charitable subscriptions of this country - for one of the Doctor's black servants (an apprentice to that great Philosopher) has actually embarked at Lancaster on board a vessel bound for the coast of Guinea; and it is whispered that he taked with him one of the Doctor's black cats. We must not therefore be surprised if, in time, we hear of "wonders! wonders! wonders!, Katterfelto and Black Cats, in the wilds of Africa!"[1]*

Perhaps the term of his indenture had come to an end and he really had set sail for Africa. Certainly, by the time Katterfelto was performing in Birmingham during 1792 he was advertising for two replacement apprentices from the indigenous community:

> *Doctor Katterfelto wants two servant Boys, about fourteen to sixteen Years of Age, from the Country or the Town; they must come from honest Families and have good Characters – They will have an Opportunity of learning the most of his various Arts and Experiments, which not one Person in ten Thousand is Master of.[2]*

Although the campaign by Wilberforce and others to outlaw the slave trade would not succeed until 1807, there was a growing (though far from universal) opposition to slavery in the country. An emphasis on human equality in social and political thought, and the growing influence of Evangelical ethics, were combining to transform the sensibility of much of the public. Had Katterfelto's moral perspective changed as well, so that out of a new conviction he let the servants go? Or had the young men simply become too much of a public liability - the cause of increasing offence among his audiences?

Perhaps the truth was that Katterfelto just could not afford to keep them any longer. With high inflation, fickle audiences, and the cost of equipment and supplies for his shows, there may not have been much money left to buy food or to replace worn out clothing for the family and servants. In addition, a decade of severe winters, poor harvests and food shortages had stretched the system of poor relief to breaking point. Parishes were increasingly reluctant to welcome vagrants who might be a burden on the public purse, making it hard for the Katterfeltos to get charitable help if they needed it. As a result, increasing financial hardship may have meant that the servants were simply discharged to fend for themselves. Or perhaps Thomas Montague and his companion finally managed to run away for good, capitalising on the increasing reluctance of the public to turn them in, and having had enough of empty stomachs and cold nights under the wagon.

It may well have been this same combination of bad weather and poor diet that made Katterfelto vulnerable to the illness that sent him on his final journey. Once again we are indebted to Hird, the shoemaker of Bedale, for the details:

> *Near twenty years, I here may say,*
> *The Doctor comes again,*
> *And then the folks, they all look'd gay,*
> *The learned were right fain!!*
> *But now he had no African,*
> *His trumpet for to blow!*
> *but he had come, the news it ran!*
> *All people soon did know!*
> *And he'd his daughter and his wife,*
> *Likewise his fine black cats!*
> *He diverted many to the life,*
> *He kept them not for rats.*
> *But he did keep them to shew skill,*
> *And shew the use of air,*
> *Which he divested at his will,*
> *As dead they did appear!!*
> *He did create a vast of fun,*
> *For some who went to see!*
> *Of models he had many a one,*
> *Which pleased the company.*
> *His paraphernalia it was great,*
> *He did it well arrange!*
> *His lectures they were quite replete,*
> *He open'd myst'rys strange!*

He always lectur'd in his gown,
All great attention paid,
His audience did all sit down,
To hear what he display'd.
Of his great loadstone he did boast!
It earn'd him many pounds!
His magnets sold at highest cost,
All over, in his rounds.
But now his time was near an end,
He sicken'd and did die!
To teach knowledge, did his life spend,
Not dreaming here to lie.
Within the church they laid him,
As they do all the great,
And there he lies, far from his kin!
Except in Adam's state.
Near t'altar steps his tomb is seen,
A plain and humble stone,
Which speaks the fame of what he'd been,
His name and age thereon.
Time when he died, and epitaph,
That's writ in four lines,
Phylosopher! That is enough!
The grave! Thy all enshrines.[3]

No doubt, in the early days of November, the topic of conversation in the little town was no longer "Have you seen his Solar Microscope Exhibition?" but "Have you heard that Katterfelto is sick?" Did any sceptics mutter "Physician heal thyself"? Neither Doctor Batto's medicines nor any of Doctor Katterfelto's own healing powers could avail him. His condition worsened and on the 15th November he passed away. He, who had set out to enlighten others so that they might know heaven's ways, would now discover whether his moral and divine philosophy had set himself on the road to God's kingdom.

However, for those left behind there was the practical matter of his funeral. The service register testifies that "William Anthony Katterfelto" was buried three days later - laid to rest in the chancel of the Church. His widow, or perhaps one or more of the residents of Bedale, paid for the grave to be covered with the "plain and humble stone" that carried the simple epitaph: "Christian William

Anthony Katterfelto, Doctor in Philosophy, died November 15th 1799, aged 56 years".[4] In a line of poetry that Hird later crossed out, he reports that the stone was subsequently covered over with floor boards, and as his editor comments: "it may well be that it still lies under the chancel floor".[5]

So why did the folks of Bedale pay Katterfelto the tribute of giving him a final resting place within their church? Seemingly for the simple reason that they believed what Katterfelto said about himself. They believed that a great philosopher had visited them, not once but twice. He had honoured them with his presence and had entertained and instructed them. Now it was their turn to honour him. Someone even paid to announce his death in the papers. On the 19th December, the York Chronicle carried the notice: "At Bedale, Yorkshire, the *wonderful* philosopher, Dr. Katterfelto", while the Gentleman's Magazine published in London, told its readers of the passing of "the eccentric Dr Katterfelto whose advertisements of himself and his black cats used, generally, to be ushered in with the word "Wonders!" three times repeated". (The magazine reports the death as occurring on the 25th November; a mistake that has frequently been repeated elsewhere.)[6]

And what of the rest of his household? Well, the cats were no longer needed for his shows but fortunately they soon found a good home: that of Mister Swann, who Hird calls the "inmate" of Bedale's Royal Oak pub. As for Mrs. and Miss Katterfelto their future was far from certain, and they may have been facing destitution. However, help, or even love, was at hand:

The widow and the daughter then,
They were of man bereft.
In Bedale, one among the men,
Eccentric! his drift.
He soon connection form'd with them,
From hence they did remove,
To Scarborough, and did remain
The object of his love!!!

The lucky man was: "John Carter, Tailor, of this parish". The church register records that he and Martha Katterfelto were married in Bedale on the 2nd March 1800. At the wedding, the widow of the great philosopher was not able to sign her own name but instead just made her mark. The marriage, coming less than four months after her husband's death, suggests that this was either a whirlwind romance or else it was a sign of Martha's rather desperate economic condition. Hird's reference to the family moving to Scarborough was probably a mistaken memory. According to the Dictionary of National Biography, Martha's new husband was the same John Carter who went on to run a pub in Whitby and to play a significant role in the development of the jet trade in that town. However, within six months of the wedding Martha was living not in Whitby but in Leeds. From the 22nd September of that year until the 12th January 1801, the Leeds Intelligencer carried the following regular announcement:

MECHANICAL MUSEUM,
With the Whole of the late Dr. KATTERFELTO's
Philosophical Apparatus,
with an Addition of the Whole of Mr. J. N. Osmond's
Natural Curiosities.
Insects to be viewed by the Large Compound Microscope.
To be seen every Day in the Week, from Ten in the Morning till
Eight at Night, (Sundays excepted) at the Museum in Vicar Lane,
Leeds - Admittance 1s.
… Magnets sold from a Guinea to a Shilling.
Six different Sorts of Phosphorus.
Likewise a New-invented Fire Machine, at 2s 6d.
A New-invented Hydgometer, to tell the Change of Weather,
at 2s 6d.
A valuable Tincture for the Tooth Ach,
which never fails curing instantly. The Bottle is 2s.
The Doctor's Widow cures Persons who are afflicted
with Nervous Disorders, Hardness of Hearing, Rheumatic Ague,
Paralytic Disorders, and such as have weak Eyes, green
Wounds, and several other Complaints.
N.B. A few Diamond Beetles, Shells, and other
Natural Curiosities, to be Sold.

Perhaps Martha and John's marriage had only lasted a few months, or maybe they had spent time together in Leeds before moving on to Whitby. Either way, whether from necessity, habit or simply the pleasure of performing, Martha Carter was trying to keep the show on the road. She had clearly kept much of her husband's equipment, exhibits and merchandise. Having already demonstrated a facility for sleights of hand in years past, it appears that she had also taken an interest in the medical side of things and was now curing people of the same complaints treated by her departed husband.

So much for Martha, but what about the children? The 1783 cartoon "The Wonderful Dr Kat-he-felt-ho" (see illustration 4) had shown Martha with a young boy at her side and carrying in her arms what looks like two young twin daughters. The absence of Mary, their eldest daughter, from the drawing may suggest that we shouldn't make too much of it - that the children are merely products of the satirist's imagination. On the other hand, perhaps this cartoon was based on knowledge of the family who had been behind the scenes, or even appeared on stage, at the London performances. If so, then the children represent Frederick William who, by now, would have been six, along with two new siblings. Nowhere else is there any reference to these other children. The young Durham lad in 1787 recalled only a daughter sitting by the fireside behind the stage curtain, just as Hird remembered only a daughter returning to Bedale in 1799. So we must surmise that, at some point on their travels, Frederick (and possibly two younger sisters) had, like so many others at the time, succumbed to a fatal childhood illness.

That the daughter who outlived her father was called Mary becomes clear on the 31st October 1833, when Mary Ann Katterfelto, spinster of the parish, was married in Leeds Parish Church. (The clergyman who conducted the service must have taken the wedding on autopilot, as Mary's wedding was one of a staggering ninety-eight that the rector and his curate conducted in October alone - a sign of the growth of the town of Leeds in this period.) And who had Mary married? It turns out to be "Jonathan Carter, Tailor, of this parish." Is it just a coincidence that Martha and Mary's two husbands shared the same surname and occupation? Could it be that stepbrother and stepsister had eventually married some thirty years after their parents?

Whatever the truth may be, Mary and Jonathan wed late in life and their marriage was to last less than seven years. They died in Leeds just three weeks apart in April and May 1840, both at the age of 70.[7] So, after spending the first thirty years of her life on the road, it seems that Mary had tired of the travelling, the stage and being raised up by magnets. She had no further interest in "wondering for her bread". Mary was content to settle down and to live out the rest of her life in Leeds. When she died Katterfelto's line came to an end. However his name still lived on.

At the start of the nineteenth century, Katterfelto's reputation for puffery was a gift to those who wanted to mock the pretensions of others. So a theatre critic in Dublin could satirise the actress Mrs. Siddons's "tragic" performance in these terms: "this Katterfelto of wonders exceeded expectation, went beyond belief and soared above all the natural powers of description!"[8] In the affairs of state the name of Katterfelto, with its associations with quackery and trickery, could be used to attack political or military opponents. The Prime Minister Henry Addington was lambasted by George Canning (who later took on the same office himself) as a quack doctor who was killing the nation. For Canning, Britain would actually be far safer facing the threat of a French invasion if it were defended, not by politicians such as Addington, but by an army of quacks including "that wonderful wonder, the great Katterfelto".[9]

On the international stage, in Henry Kirke White's song "The Wonderful Juggler", Napoleon Bonaparte found himself described as "this new Katterfelto", because of the belief that he would trick his way past the British fleet using ships that could travel under water.[10] On a more local level, in 1803 a political satire in the form of a theatre bill appeared in Hereford lampooning the unopposed election of a new Member of Parliament, who had previously been a doctor of medicine. It suggested that the new MP was none other than "Katterfelto redivivus": the "Wonderful Wonder of Wonders" who had borrowed the ninth life of his black cat in order to arise from the grave.[11] The political interest in him continued through the nineteenth century. In 1836 Benjamin Disraeli, writing under a pseudonym in The Times, ridiculed the Chancellor of the Exchequer as "you and your Katterfelto crew".[12] Even in the early years of the twentieth century there were still references to "political Katterfelto quackery".[13]

The epitome of quackery was also remembered on occasions by some in the medical profession. One doctor, Matthew Lewis, was reminded of him when living and working on a slave plantation in the West Indies. He wrote that, "In my medical capacity I sometimes perform cures so unexpected, that I stand like Katterfelto 'with my hair standing on end at my wonders',"[14] (an allusion to Cowper's poem that was copied by many). Travellers in America who encountered wonder-working mountebanks named them "Katterfelto"[15] or remembered him as "the by-gone professor of legerdemain".[16]

His name entered into several works of fiction, most notably

171

Whyte-Melville's 1875 novel: "Katerfelto". In this, "the celebrated Doctor Katerfelto" is the villain of the piece. He is portrayed as a charlatan and "the devil in person", of whom it could be said that "no man alive had fewer scruples of mercy or forbearance". Despite this, he provides treatment to another character, John Garnet, who names his Exmoor horse after the doctor; a horse that was remarkable for its speed and endurance. The idea for this had come to Whyte-Melville when he was researching his novel on a hunting trip to Exmoor. Here he learnt of "Katerfelto", a stallion that had wandered the moor around sixty years earlier. It is not clear whether the horse was mythical or real, but several other horses on Exmoor were later given the same name, and many of the New Forest ponies are said to descend from one of these. No doubt it was the speed of the famous stallion (it certainly wasn't the speed of our hero) that led the Great Western Railway to christen one of its engines, "Katerfelto". As for the Doctor's connection to the dark arts, Whyte-Melville and Roget's Thesaurus were not the only ones to preserve this association. In our own day, the Romanian Branch of "The Great European Pentagramma" claims Katterfelto as one of their own: that is, as a vampire![17]

His skills as a magician were recorded in some detail by Thomas Frost in the pioneering 1876 work, "The Lives of the Conjurors". (Frost also wrote about Breslaw, although he dismissed Boaz as one of "the small fry of the profession".)[18] In addition, unlike almost all of his conjuring rivals and peers, Katterfelto's name lived on in the popular imagination. However, part of his name didn't. Somewhere along the way, Christian William Anthony Katterfelto has become known as "Gustavus Katterfelto" in all modern references to him. How did this happen?

We might assume that Gustavus was simply his stage name, and yet never once did he use a first name in any of his advertisements. Likewise, those who wrote about him when he was alive followed his own lead and simply called him "Katterfelto". The same is true after his death: his entry in Stephen Jones's "Biographical Dictionary", which first appeared in Katterfelto's lifetime but the final version of which was published in 1840, lacks any reference to a first name.

The man responsible for publicly christening Katterfelto as "Gustavus" turns out to be someone born thirty-eight years after his death: a solicitor from Cambridge by the name of Thompson Cooper. Thompson had followed his father Charles into the legal profession, but the census record for 1861 shows that they both also considered themselves to be authors.[19] Thompson was working on "A New Dictionary of Biography" and two years later he was doing some research for it in Whitby. Here, people with long memories and longer lives (or maybe their children) had told him tales of the philosopher-magician who had visited their town on several occasions; how he had lifted his daughter up by a magnet; and how his widow and her new husband had moved to Whitby after their wedding. They had also been able to give Katterfelto a first name.

Cooper published his findings in a newspaper article in the town in 1863,[20] although sadly no copies of it have survived. However, he went on to incorporate this information into his dictionary which was published in 1883. Here, for the first time in print, eighty-four years after Katterfelto's death, we find him called "Gustavus". Was the name that Thompson Cooper had heard on the streets of Whitby an accurate memory of a stage name? We will never know. What we do know is that the name stuck and has been associated with him ever since. Doubtless Katterfelto wouldn't have minded either way. It all adds a little bit more to his mystique.

Even if he got it wrong, we are indebted to Cooper. In 1892, his article on Katterfelto appeared almost verbatim in the National Dictionary of Biography, thus ensuring that the memory of the prince of puff was preserved and propagated well into the twentieth century. On the other hand, Cooper made no mention of Katterfelto's rivals, Breslaw or Boaz, and so neither did the National Dictionary. This alone would have made Katterfelto smile. However, he would have been even happier to know that his wish had been granted: his name had indeed lasted a hundred years. Two centuries on he must be smiling still.

---

[1] 2nd June 1790, The Cumberland Pacquet
[2] 16th July 1792, Aris's Birmingham Gazette
[3] Hird's Annal's of Bedale, op cit, pages 221-2
[4] Hird's Annals of Bedale, op cit, page 233
[5] Hird's Annals of Bedale, op cit, page 223
[6] The Gentleman's Magazine, volume 69, December 1799
[7] See the funeral entries on 27th April 1840 and 19th May 1840, St Mark's Church, Woodhouse, Leeds.
[8] Quoted by John S Adams, "Town and Country", chapter 203, 1893
[9] The Grand Consulation, George Canning
[10] "The Wonderful Juggler" in "The Poetical Works of Henry Kirke White", by Henry Kirke White

[11] Held at Hereford Museum

[12] The Runnymede Letters, Letter 6, 1836

[13] In "Wanted-A Race fit for War" by Dr. T. Miller Maguire, in "The New Age: a weekly review of politics, literature, and art", no. 732, 19th September 1908

[14] Journal of a Residence among the Negroes of the West Indies, entry for 23rd April 1818

[15] Edwin James's Account of SH Long's Expedition, Volume 5, chapter 2

[16] John Benwell, "An Englishman's Travels in America", chapter 3, 1857

[17] www.morgom.com/livros/Manual%20Pratico%20de%20 Vampirismo.pdf

[18] Thomas Frost, op cit, chapter 6

[19] See the 1861 census for Cambridge

[20] 11th December 1863, Whitby Times

FOLLOWING IN KATTERFELTO'S FOOTSTEPS

Below is a detailed itinerary of Katterfelto's travels. Inevitably there are gaps. The larger of these are usually during periods when he was travelling through areas not covered by local newspapers, or where the newspapers have not survived. Other gaps reflect the fact that the smaller towns he visited are rarely mentioned in the advertisements. However, when these do appear it is clear just how thoroughly he covered many areas of the country. In a few cases the locations quoted reflect Katterfelto's expressed intention to visit them, although whether he actually arrived cannot be confirmed. (These are marked with an asterisk.)

A long period of uncertainty is the years from 1777 to 1780. However, Katterfelto's publicity material at the end of this time is more or less the same as it was at the start. The greater variety and creativity of his advertisements and his shows seems to have developed during his years in London.

Usually, the dates for his stays in any town or city are not precise. He sometimes gives the date of his arrival but almost never gives us information about exactly when he will be leaving. When a single date is given in the itinerary this indicates the date of a single advert but does not imply that Katterfelto only performed there for one day. For all its incompleteness, what emerges is an astonishing journey: twenty-three years of continuous travelling and performing around Britain.

The itinerary is followed by a list of the newspapers and their abbreviations that have been used as sources. Tracing Katterfelto's journey and telling his story has involved delving into the fascinating world of eighteenth century newspapers. Fortunately most of these survive, although once again there are gaps. For those tempted to delve into these newspapers, in search of Katterfelto or just to explore this age of wonders, the best way to begin is through the website of the British Library. Here there are links to "Newsplan", a remarkable online catalogue detailing precisely which newspapers are held by which libraries. The single largest collection is at the British Library's Collindale branch, while the British Library at St. Pancras holds an extensive collection of papers mainly from London, called the Burney Collection. However, the libraries of most cities and some towns have a collection of local papers from the period. The papers can usually only be read on microfilm, but occasionally the hard copies are available, which is a real treat.

DATE	LOCATION	VENUE	SOURCE
1776			
Sep 26th-Sep 3th	Hull	Concert Room	YC
Oct 8th-Oct 27th	York	Nicholson's Great Room, Coney Street	YC
Oct 28th - Nov 5th	Leeds		YC
	Wakefield*		YC
	Halifax*		YC
	Bedale (between 1776-80)		Hird's Annals

1777

Nov 24th - Nov 30th	Gloucester	George's Coffe House, West Gate Street	GJ

1780

Dec 9th	Arrives London		MH
Dec 9th - May 1781		Great Room, Spring Gardens	MC,MH, MP

1781

May 2nd - Jun 13th		228 High Holborn	MC
Jun 13th	Ends 'Season'		MC

1782

Feb 26th - Apr 14th		Great Room, Spring Gardens	MC, MH, MP
Apr 15th - Feb 1783		22, Piccadily	GA, MC, MH. MP

1783

Feb 19th - Jul 1784		24, Piccadily	GA, MC, MH, MP

1784

c. Jul 13th	Leaves London		MP etc
Aug 21st - Sep 4th	Colchester	Town Hall	IJ
Sep 9th - Sep 18th	Ipswich	The Council Chamber, Town Hall	IJ

	Bury (St. Edmonds)		NC
Nov 27th - Jan 22nd 1785	Norwich	Exhibition Room, Rampant Horse Street	NoC

1785

Jun 10th	(Kings) Lynn	The Duke's Head	CC
Jul 9th - Aug 6th	Wisbech	The Rose and Crown	CC
Aug 20th	Northampton		CC
Sep 14th - Sep 17th	Stamford	The George and Angel	CC
	Peterborough*		CC
Oct 7th – Oct 12th	Spalding		LRSM
Nov 4th - Nov 25th	Boston	Assembly Room, Town Hall	LRSM

Jan 18th	Lincoln		LRSM
Feb 7th–Feb 20th	Grantham		LRSM
	Newark*		LRSM
	Gainsborough*		LRSM
	Sheffield		ISA (1796)
Oct 5th	Beverley		YCh¹
Oct 9th - Oct 12th	IIull		YC
Nov 28th	Pontefract		LM
Dec 3rd–Dec 8th	Nostell Priory		LI
Dec 9th–Dec 21st	Leeds	Old Assembly Room, Kirkgate	LI + LM
Dec 22nd–mid Jan 1787	York	Mr Grice's large room, Stonegate and a Private House, Bootham Bar	YC

	Richmond		NC
Mar 31st	Northallerton		NC
Apr 20th	Durham		NC
May 3rd	Sunderland	George Inn	NC
May 29th - Jun 20th	Newcastle	St. John's Lodge, Low Friar Street	NC
Jul 6th - Jul 21st	North Shields		NC
Aug 13th - Aug 21st	Berwick (on Tweed)	Town Hall	EA + CM
early Sep	Haddington	Town Hall	EA
Oct 9th - Feb 2nd 1788	Edinburgh	Dunn's Hotel, New Town (Solar Microscope) Craig's Close, High Street (Lectures) No. 3, St Andrew Street, New Town	EA+ CM

1788

	St Andrews*		CM
	Perth*		CM
Jun 10th - Jul 8th	Dundee	Trade's Hall	AJ
Jul 15th - Jul 29th	Montrose		AJ
Aug 9th - Aug 18th	Aberdeen	St Nicholas's Hall, Queen Street staying at the New Inn	AJ
	Peterhead*		AJ
Aug 23rd- Aug 28th	Banff		AJ
	Elgin*		AJ
	Nairn*		AJ
	Inverness*		AJ

1789

Mar 6th	Glasgow	Black Bull Inn	Bell Geordie[2]
Jun 2nd-Aug 7th	Glasgow	Frazer's Hall, King Street	GAEI + GM Bell Geordie[3]
	Kilmarnock*		GAEI
	Ayr*		GAEI
Nov 24th	Dumfries		DGS
Dec 7th-Dec 30th	Carlisle	Council Room, Town Hall	CP

	Maryport		CP
Jan 13th- Jan 20th	Cockermouth	Assembly Room	CP
Jan 27th - Mar 17th	Whitehaven	Globe Inn, Howgill Street (Solar Microscope) Assembly Room, Howgill Street (Evening Lecture) The Old Sugar House, Duke St (Wonders)	CP
	Workington*		CP
	Keswick*		CP
	Penrith		CP
Apr	Appleby*		CP
May 1st - May 6th	Kendal		CP
May 13th - Jun 2nd	Lancaster		CP
Jul 6th - Aug 10th	Manchester	The Exchange	MM

1791

Jan 5th - Jan 21st	Chester	House next to Golden Lion, Foregate Street	CC
	Wrexham		SC (1793)
Mar 1st - Mar 2nd	Warrington		WLA
Mar 14th - May 2nd	Liverpool	The Golden Lion, Dale Street Home of Hon. T. Fitzmaurice, Marble street	WLA
	Knutsford*		CC
	Congleton*		CC
Sept 28th	Newcastle-u-Lyme	Town Hall	WC
Nov 22nd - Nov 30th	Stafford		WC + ABG
Dec 21st - late Jan 1792	Wolverhampton	Old Bell Inn	WC + ABG

1792

Feb	Willenhall		ABG
	Wednesford		ABG
	Bilston		ABG
	Walsall*		WC
Feb 27th - Apr 2nd	Dudley	Town Hall	ABG
	Stourbridge*		WC
Apr 9th	arrives Brimingham	32 New Street	ABG

1793

post Apr 1st	Leaves Birmingham		ABG
	Arley Hall		SC
Sep 6th - Oct 18th	Shrewsbury	White Lion Inn, Raven Street	SC
Nov 26th	Oswestry		SC
	Ellesmere		SC

1794

Jun 16th - Jul 2nd	Ludlow	Assembly Room, Town Hall	HJ
Jul 31st	Leominster		HJ
Aug 13th - Sep 11th	Hereford	Preece's Assembly or Coffee Room The Theatre	HJ
Nov 9th - 25th	Monmouth	Town Hall (Grand Exhibition) Beaufort Arms (Solar Microscope)	GJ
Dec 15th - Feb 2nd 1795	Gloucester	The New Inn	GJ

1795

Apr 23rd - Jun 4th	Worcester	Old Assembly Room, The Bull Inn, Broad Street	BWJ
Jul 6th	Bromsgrove		ABG
Sep 7th	Lichfield	Vicar's Hall	ABG
Oct 15th - late Dec	Derby	The Talbot Inn	DM

1796

Jan 9th - Apr 16th	Nottingham	The Great Room, Grindlesmith-gate (Solar Microscope) The Exchange, or Thurland Hall (evening) Tickets from Backmoor's Head. Staying at Spread Eagle Inn, Long Row	NJ
	Mansfield		ISA
Jun 14th - Mid Jul	Chesterfield		ISA
Jul 30th- Sep 27th	Sheffield	Freemason's Lodge, Paradise Square, Howard Street	ISA & ShC

1797

Jan 9th - Mar 20th	York	White Dog Inn, Stonegate	YC & YH

1798

Aug 20th - Aug 25th	Sunderland		NC
Sep 8th - Dec 9th	Newcastle	Philosophical Society Room in St Nicholas's Churchyard	NC

1799

Nov 15th	Bedale		Hird's Annals

---

[1] University of Hull Library Archives, ref DX173/9

[2] www.amostcuriousmurder.com/BellGeordie.htm mistakenly dated as 1787

[3] "Dr Katterfelto, that great divine and moral philosopher, is now about to exhibit again in this city

ABBREVIATIONS OF NEWSPAPER TITLES

ABG	Aris's Birmingham Gazette
AJ	The Aberdeen Journal
BC	The Bath Chronicle
BG	The Bristol Gazette and Public Advertiser
BWJ	Berrow's Worcester Journal
CaC	The Cambridge Chronicle
ChC	The Chester Chronicle
CM	The Caledonian Mercury (Edinburgh)
CP	The Cumberland Pacquet and Ware's Whitehaven Advertiser
DA	The Daily Advertiser (London)
DGS	Dumfries and Galloway Standard
DM	The Derby Mercury
EA	The Edinburgh Advertiser
EEC	The Edinburgh Evening Courant
FFBJ	Felix Farley's Bristol Journal
GA	The General Advertiser (London)
GAEI	The Glasgow Advertiser and Evening Intelligencer
GJ	The Gloucester Journal
GM	The Glasgow Mercury
HJ	The Hereford Journal
IJ	The Ipswich Journal
ISA	The Iris or Sheffield Advertiser
KC	The Kelso Chronicle
LC	The London Courant
LM	The Leeds Mercury
LI	The Leeds Intelligencer
LRSM	The Lincoln, Rutland and Stamford Mercury
MC	The Morning Chronicle and London Advertiser
MH	The Morning Herald and Daily Advertiser (London)
MM	The Manchester Mercury and Harrop's General Advertiser

MP	The Morning Post and Daily Advertiser (London)
NC	The Newcastle Courant
NoC	The Norfolk Chronicle
NJ	The Nottingham Journal
SC	The Shrewsbury Chronicle
ShC	The Sheffield Courant
WC	The Wolverhampton Chronicle
WLA	Williamson's Liverpool Advertiser and Marine Intelligencer
YCh	The York Chronicle
YC	The York Courant
YH	The York Herald
YJ	The Yorkshire Journal (Doncaster)

INDEX

195